# SpringerBriefs in Public Health

W0227835

For further volumes:
http://www.springer.com/series/10138

Seth C. Kalichman

# HIV Treatments as Prevention (TasP)

Primer for Behavior-Based Implementation

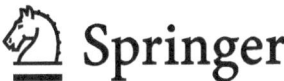 Springer

Seth C. Kalichman
Center for HIV Intervention and Prevention
University of Connecticut
Storrs, CT, USA

ISSN 2192-3698                  ISSN 2192-3701 (electronic)
ISBN 978-1-4614-5118-1          ISBN 978-1-4614-5119-8 (eBook)
DOI 10.1007/978-1-4614-5119-8
Springer New York Heidelberg Dordrecht London

Library of Congress Control Number: 2012944180

Printed on acid-free paper

Springer is part of Springer Science+Business Media (www.springer.com)

# Preface

Because HIV is contracted only through a few specific behaviors, AIDS is a completely preventable disease. This simple fact motivates the field of AIDS behavioral research. Ultimately, our efforts are geared toward developing and testing interventions. Unfortunately, our interventions have only had a few tools to leverage against the virus. The good news in HIV prevention is that our toolbox is expanding. But with these new opportunities come new challenges. This Brief offers my perspective on using antiretroviral treatments as the latest tool for prevention. I am specifically interested in how behavioral interventions will be integrated with antiretroviral medications to prevent people living with HIV from transmitting the virus. The same medications can keep uninfected people from becoming infected, but this Brief is not concerned with pre-exposure prophylaxis (PrEP). The opportunities and challenges facing PrEP are different and warrant their own attention.

The idea for this Brief came from nearly a decade of AIDS behavioral research. My research team has been interested in developing interventions to reduce sexual risk behaviors in people living with HIV. Our first attempt demonstrated promising results. That intervention was subsequently packaged by the CDC as *Healthy Relationships,* which has been implemented by hundreds of providers around the USA. *Healthy Relationships* has also been adapted for use in Russia, South Africa, Botswana, and perhaps elsewhere. After completing *Healthy Relationships*, we worked on interventions to improve HIV treatment adherence. It was apparent that the obstacles to medication adherence were the same as those for sexual risk reduction—moods, motivation, stigma, disclosure, social environments, and substance use. In fact, the interventions we developed for medication adherence were based on the same theoretical models as *Healthy Relationships*. It became clear that these interventions could be integrated to simultaneously reduce HIV transmission risks and improve medication adherence. We therefore developed an integrated model for HIV prevention and treatment adherence called *In the Mix*. Our experience with *In the Mix* builds a foundation for this Brief.

Storrs, CT, USA                                                                                       Seth C. Kalichman

# Acknowledgments

There are many who have contributed to this work. Lisa Eaton at the University of Connecticut fueled many of these ideas. Lisa always knows the right questions to ask and she is the most resourceful person I have known when it comes to finding the right answers. Without Lisa's collaborations I am quite sure my work would have stayed stuck in the 1990s. I am also fortunate to have a team of dedicated researchers working on our interventions; Chauncey Cherry, Demetria Cain, Moira Kalichman, Christina Amaral, Tamar Grebler, Denise White, Mich'l Jones, Megan McNerney, Ginger Hoyt, Cindy Merley, Brandi Welles, Daniel Driffin, Harlan Smith, and Jennie Pellowski. I am also grateful to the National Institutes of Health for supporting our prevention and adherence research. This Brief would never have been completed without the support of Bill Tucker at Springer Science. Bill is everything I could ask for in an Editor. I am forever grateful to him. Finally, this Brief is dedicated to the memory of HIV Treatment Advocate Dan Dunable and to the future of Hannah Kalichman. Both Dan and Hannah remain my most enduring sources of inspiration.

# Contents

# Chapter 1
# Foundations and Principles

*Yet today, here we are, talking seriously about the "end" of this global epidemic. There are now 6.6 million people on life-saving AIDS medicine. But still too many are being infected. New research proves that early antiretroviral treatment, especially for pregnant women, in combination with male circumcision, will slash the rate of new H.I.V. cases by up to 60 percent. This is the tipping point we have been campaigning for. We're nearly there.*

*Bono, The New York Times, November 30, 2011 (Available at http://www.nytimes.com/2011/12/01/opinion/a-decade-of-progress-on-aids.html)*

HIV prevention has pivoted away from focusing on those uninfected toward identifying people infected with the virus and treating them with antiretroviral therapies. Although it may seem odd that prevention relies on those already afflicted with the disease to stop the spread of HIV, the history of AIDS makes clear how we got here. The first significant breakthrough in AIDS prevention came in the diagnostic revolution, which occurred in 1985 following the advent of HIV antibody tests. With the test, people were able to learn whether they had been infected with HIV. The test also allowed for meaningful measures to protect the public health, namely screening the blood supply. Combining testing technologies for various HIV antibodies and antigens has brought greater sensitivities and specificities to diagnosing HIV infection. Diagnostic testing was also combined with risk reduction counseling, which became the universal driving force in the fight against the spread of HIV. A decade later, in 1996, came the second revolution—this time in HIV treatments. It was easy to make the case against testing before there were effective treatments. After all, what is the value in knowing your HIV status in the absence of effective treatments? Combinations of antiretroviral medications suppress viral replication, effectively slowing the HIV disease process. However, effective HIV treatment is not always easy to attain. Antiretroviral therapy is expensive and requires strict long-term adherence.

More than 30 years into the AIDS epidemic, we are now in the midst of a third revolution—the prevention revolution. Like the diagnostic and treatment revolutions of the past, the prevention revolution is fueled by multiple strategies that, when used in combinations, have the potential to surpass the effects of any one approach. The first 30 years of AIDS have given us dozens of behavioral prevention

S.C. Kalichman, *HIV Treatments as Prevention (TasP):*
*Primer for Behavior-Based Implementation*, SpringerBriefs in Public Health,
DOI 10.1007/978-1-4614-5119-8_1, © Seth C. Kalichman 2013

interventions delivered at individual, couple, group, and community levels. However, no single intervention is completely protective and all require maintenance to achieve long-term behavior change. Now we have available a growing arsenal of biological prevention technologies, which for the most part, are also not completely protective and require long-term behavior change.

Our task in the prevention revolution is therefore to find the right combinations of biomedical and behavioral interventions for maximum impact. The key to success will be synergism. Just as an ELISA antibody test must be combined with Western Blot to diagnose HIV and just as using AZT alone can do more harm than good, prevention requires multi-strategy approaches. Fortunately, years of investment in behavioral research has yielded a wealth of information about how to optimally market, engage, implement, and sustain preventive behaviors.

In the early days of the AIDS epidemic, prevention concentrated on disseminating information about how HIV causes AIDS and how people do and do not contract HIV. Grassroots organizations in major US cities, particularly Gay Men's Health Crisis and Stop AIDS San Francisco, developed what would become model programs for organizing and mobilizing outreach to those most at-risk for HIV. These pioneers in prevention invented the AIDS risk reduction workshop that brought community members together to discuss AIDS and ways to stay safe [1]. Word spread and AIDS education workshops and community forums sprung-up around the country.

The widespread dissemination of understandable and accessible information clearly had an impact. Studies show that gay men increased their condom use, reduced their numbers of sex partners, and sought HIV testing. Similarly, injection drug users learned how to disinfect their needles and syringes, and refrained from sharing injection equipment. But not everyone at-risk changed his or her behavior. In the second decade of AIDS, prevention messages shifted from educational to fear inducing. It soon became apparent that those who were resistant to both education and fear messages would require more intensive approaches.

The next generation of prevention relied on risk reduction counseling and skills building workshops. These interventions focused on individual needs, motivations, and behavioral self-management skills. Intensive behavior change interventions were rooted in techniques drawn from cognitive-behavioral therapy, emphasizing coping, problem solving, decision-making, social influences, motivational enhancement, behavioral rehearsal, feedback, planning, and reinforcement. With overwhelming evidence, these interventions effectively reduced syringe-mediated and sexually transmitted infections (STI). Significant strides in behavioral interventions were made despite committing the vast majority of HIV prevention resources to vaccine development.

## Behavioral Interventions

There was substantial evidence as early as 1997 that behavioral interventions can prevent the spread of HIV. An expert panel convened by the National Institutes of Health (NIH) to find consensus on the state of HIV prevention science concluded that training people with drug addictions in safer injection practices was without question effective in preventing HIV infections (available at http://consensus.nih.gov/1997/19 97PreventHIVRisk104PDF.pdf). The Consensus Panel also found compelling evidence for the effectiveness of community outreach, risk reduction counseling, and small group cognitive-behavioral risk reduction workshops. The Panel stated:

> Three approaches are particularly effective for risk in drug abuse behavior: needle exchange programs, drug abuse treatment, and outreach programs for drug abusers not enrolled in treatment. Several programs were deemed effective for risky sexual behavior. These programs include (a) information about HIV/AIDS and (b) building skills to use condoms and to negotiate the interpersonal challenges of safer sex. Effective safer sex programs have been developed for men who have sex with men, for women, and for adolescents.... Because behavioral interventions are currently the only effective way of slowing the spread of HIV infection, recommendations coming from this conference have immediate implications for service delivery in health care and educational settings, including schools; substance abuse treatment programs; community-based organizations; sexually transmitted disease clinics; inner-city health programs reaching disenfranchised high-risk women, men, and adolescents; rural health programs; and mental health programs that serve high-risk people with chronic mental illness.

Success was also evident at the population level. In Thailand, for example, the government instituted what became known as the 100% condom campaign [2]. The program included mandatory condom use by commercial sex workers, provided free condoms to sex workers, and introduced a mass advertising campaign to promote condom use. Between 1989 and 1993 condom use increased from 14 to 94% of commercial sex acts. In 1992 alone the government supplied 45 million condoms to commercial sex establishments, protecting an estimated 79% of commercial sex acts, with the private sector supplying enough additional condoms to protect 126% of all commercial sex acts. Trends in STI clinic visits tracked the program's implementation. Between 1989 and 1993 gonorrhea declined 85% and other STI declined 74%.

HIV prevention success was also observed in Uganda, where 30% reduction in HIV prevalence occurred among women seeking pregnancy services in some of the hardest hit areas of the country [3]. HIV reductions were even greater among younger women. National HIV prevalence was near 30% in the early 1990s and astonishingly dropped to 7%. Gary Slutkin, who worked for the World Health Organization on AIDS prevention in Uganda during the 1990s attributes the success to an influx of international support for HIV prevention, stating:

> Uganda developed the first, and what was soon to become, the strongest planned and best supported National AIDS Program, with the largest national and international staffing and most intensive, broadly inclusive, decentralized and community based public education program in Africa. When Uganda was receiving $18 million in support, other countries in the region were receiving between $1 million to $4 million. External and national financial support to the Uganda program was 4–20 times the amount provided to any other national program outside of the industrialized world at the time [4].

Mike Merson was head of the WHO's Global AIDS Program at the time, and he amplifies Slutkin's observations, further stating:

> The prevention success of Uganda is thus attributable to the provision of full information about all means of transmission and protection by many sectors of society, along with efforts to destigmatize HIV/AIDS by being open about the disease, showing compassion

and providing care to those who are infected and affected. Those who are skeptical about the potential effectiveness of behavior change programs need to realize what the Uganda experience tells us, namely that these programs can only be successful if they are comprehensive, well funded, and given the priority that today is being awarded to treatment with antiretroviral drugs [5].

In the absence of sustained efforts to maintain gains, prevention successes can be short lived. In Uganda, there remain over 110,000 new HIV infections every year. At a news conference in Entebbe in 2011, Dr. Wuhib Tadesse Director of CDC-Uganda stated that HIV prevention in Uganda has stagnated, threatening to reverse what has been a prevention success. While several factors are likely at play in Uganda's HIV epidemic, complacency appears at least partly to blame for lost ground. Without plans for comprehensive, ongoing, sustained, and agile prevention programming, it is doubtful that any prevention strategy will succeed in the long term.

## The HIV Prevention Toolbox

Advances in HIV prevention have occurred at the cellular, behavioral, dyadic, network, family, and community levels. Table 1.1 shows the levels of HIV prevention and a summary of evidence for interventions in each level. I define definitive success when the intervention has demonstrated efficacy in at least one randomized clinical trial with an objective-disease relevant outcome. Interventions that have yielded inconsistent findings across randomized trials are defined as mixed. Interventions that lack positive outcomes are considered poor. I rely on randomized trials because they ultimately provide the most convincing evidence for efficacy. Of course, the status of any intervention approach is subject to change as new trials are completed. Rigorous prevention trials and systematic reviews reveal numerous successful strategies available for HIV prevention. HIV is more difficult to transmit than most other blood borne and sexually transmitted pathogens. Extrapolating intervention effects to proxy diseases such as Hepatitis C in injection drug users and STI in sexual risk populations is reasonable. Interventions that demonstrate reductions in self-reported sexual behaviors or drug use practices should not be discarded, but they are several steps away from claiming victory in preventing HIV infections.

Interventions targeted to multiple levels have met stringent standards for demonstrating definitive evidence for preventing HIV transmission. At the cellular level condoms, male circumcision, treating HIV-infected persons, and using HIV treatments for preexposure prophylaxis have shown definitive evidence for preventing HIV transmission. Unfortunately cervical protection, vaccines, and microbicides have not been so successful. The search for an effective HIV vaccine has thus far proven futile. In addition, more than 20 years of vaginal gels that were hoped to prevent HIV transmission have failed to do so. In some cases, vaccines and microbicides have even increased the risks for HIV transmission [6].

Also at the cellular level, STI treatments aimed to prevent HIV infections have delivered mixed results. One major study conducted in Malawi in the 1990s showed

**Table 1.1** Levels of HIV prevention interventions and summary of intervention effectiveness

| Level | Mechanism | Preventive intervention | Effectiveness |
|---|---|---|---|
| Cellular | Infectiousness, susceptibility | Condoms | Definitive |
| | | Antiretroviral therapy | Definitive |
| | | Male circumcision | Definitive |
| | | Preexposure treatment | Definitive |
| | | Cervical protection | Mixed |
| | | STI treatment | Mixed |
| | | Microbicides | Mixed |
| | | Vaccines | Poor |
| Individual behavior | Exposure behaviors, cognitive and emotional states, decisions, preferences, addictions | Risk reduction counseling | Definitive |
| | | Prevention workshops | Definitive |
| | | Addiction treatment | Mixed |
| | | Mental health counseling | Poor |
| Dyadic/couples | Relationships, power dynamics, love, affection | Couples counseling | Mixed |
| | | Couples testing | Mixed |
| Networks | Social relations Sexual relations Needle sharing relations | Sex network behavior change | Definitive |
| | | Injection behavior change | Definitive |
| Family | Family support | Parental monitoring | Poor |
| | | Family counseling | Poor |
| Institutions | Schools, places of worship, clinics, bars and clubs, shooting galleries | Comprehensive sex education | Mixed |
| | | Venue-based STI screening | Mixed |
| | | Drinking venue interventions | Mixed |
| | | Drug venue interventions | Mixed |
| | | Abstinence programs | Mixed |
| | | Faith-based program | Poor |
| Communities | Neighborhoods, cities, cyberspace | Community mobilization | Definitive |
| | | Social marketing | Mixed |
| | | Peer outreach | Mixed |
| | | Opinion leaders | Mixed |
| | | Internet interventions | Mixed |
| Structural | Policies Laws Social structures | Syringe access | Definitive |
| | | Needle exchange | Definitive |
| | | Access to care/treatment | Mixed |
| | | Disclosure criminalization | Poor |
| | | Sodomy laws | Poor |
| | | Oppressive drug laws | Poor |

that treating STI through comprehensive services reduced HIV incidence. However, a subsequent study conducted in Rakai Uganda failed to show that a more limited approach to treating STI prevents HIV infections. Observation studies show promising effects of suppressing Herpes Simplex Virus for reducing HIV shedding in the genital tract [7]. But randomized trials have tested treatments for herpes simplex virus infection, the major source of genital ulcerations, with disappointing results [8, 9]. Given that STI are a significant cofactor for HIV infectivity, it is surprising that STI treatments have not shown definitive evidence for reducing HIV transmission. One reason may be poor adherence. Failing to complete STI treatment, or maintaining adherence to herpes suppressing medications, will undermine the preventive benefits of STI treatment.

At the level of an individual's behavior, risk reduction counseling and workshops have consistently demonstrated reductions in sexual and drug use risks, making them among the most promising interventions for HIV prevention. In addition, several models aimed at reducing individual risk reduction have demonstrated clear and compelling efficacy in preventing STI and HIV transmission. On the other hand, drug treatment programs have shown mixed results for preventing HIV. Aside from the reductions in risk that come from not injecting drugs, behavior change is more likely when individuals are sober. Breaking away from drug using networks where HIV prevalence is likely high will also reduce risks. Drug treatment has a critical place in the prevention of HIV transmission and drug treatment programs offer an efficient vehicle for delivering effective prevention interventions.

Fewer prevention trials have been conducted with couples, families, and communities. Risk reduction interventions for couples demonstrate mixed results with some studies in southern Africa demonstrating reductions in STI following couples HIV counseling and testing. However, the largest behavioral intervention for HIV serodiscordant couples, the Eban Trial, increased protective sexual risk behaviors, but did not prevent STI or HIV infections [10]. Network level interventions have proven effective in reducing injection drug and sexual behavior risks, including reductions in STI. The key to HIV prevention is therefore the integration of multiple partially effective prevention strategies. Combining prevention interventions to create maximally effective packages is indeed the future of HIV prevention. However, it remains uncertain what interventions will be optimal and feasible to combine. Behavioral interventions have thus far been included in every combination of HIV prevention packages. Why the universal inclusion of behavioral interventions? It is because failure to address social and behavioral aspects of risk invariably undermines every partially protective prevention technology.

## Behavior Trumps Biology

David Bangsberg at Harvard Medical School has pointed out that behavior trumps biology in HIV prevention. Years before any study had proven the concept, Bangsberg foresaw the potential impact of antiretroviral-based prevention, but said the trick would be maintaining adequate levels of adherence necessary for protection. Distribution, access, uptake, education, and perhaps most critically adherence will dictate the impact of HIV treatments for prevention.

Along with adherence, behavioral risk compensation also trumps biology. Even slight population level changes in condom use, which seem inevitable given anti-condom sentiments, can offset the protective benefits of otherwise effective strategies [11, 12]. Mathematical modeling shows that every biomedical prevention technology requires stable patterns of behavior over time to achieve prevention goals. When people feel safer and let down their guard the result is simply less protection.

Poor adherence and heightened risk compensation therefore have the potential to diminish the value of using HIV treatment as prevention (TasP). Martin Fishbein is another visionary who saw biomedical interventions coming years before the results of any successful biomedical prevention trials. He also discussed how behavior trumps biology in HIV prevention when the only biomedical prevention technologies available were condoms, needles, and testing. In a presentation to the 1997 NIH Consensus Development Conference on Interventions to Prevent HIV Risk Behaviors, Fishbein illustrated how behavior directly impacts HIV infectivity by using May and Anderson's 1987 reproductive model of sexual HIV transmission. May and Anderson showed that the sexual reproductive rate of HIV can be represented as

$$Ro = \beta cD.$$

where $Ro =$ the reproductive rate (of transmission), $\beta =$ measure of infectivity or transmissibility, $c =$ measure of interaction between the susceptible and infected partners, and $D =$ a measure of duration of infectiousness. Fishbein used this model as a springboard, from which he went on to illustrate the following:

Because each of the elements in the right side of the equation can be influenced by behavior change, the model suggests that there are many behaviors that affect the rate of HIV transmission. For example, the degree of infectivity or transmissibility ($\beta$) can be decreased by increasing condom use or by delaying the onset of sexual activity. The interaction rate ($c$) can be influenced by decreasing the rate of new partner acquisition or increasing monogamy. Although there is no way at present to change the duration of infectiousness ($D$) for HIV, it should be noted that sexually transmitted diseases (STDs) serve as co-factors in HIV transmission (i.e., they influence $\beta$) and duration of infectiousness ($D$) is a very important parameter in reducing the transmission of STDs. Thus, if one can increase the likelihood that people will participate in screening or if they can be motivated to seek early treatment for symptomatic STDs, this will reduce the duration of infectiousness ($D$) for an STD, which ultimately reduces seroincidence.

If an effective behavioral intervention (e.g., one leading to a 15 percent increase in condom use) is introduced in a population that has low HIV prevalence, there may be little or no impact on disease. However, such an intervention could lower the probability of an epidemic if HIV were introduced into that low-prevalence population; persons would already have been inoculated (behaviorally) against the threat of HIV if at some point HIV were introduced into the social system. Yet this same intervention could have a dramatic impact on HIV seroincidence if it were introduced in a population with high seroprevalence.

Clearly, the impact of any given behavior change (like the impact of any STD control program) will depend on many factors, not the least of which is the prevalence rate of the disease in the population under consideration. Although it is possible to model the effects of a given increase in condom use (or decrease in STDs) on the HIV epidemic, it is important to recognize that the same 10 or 15 percent increase in condom use (or reduction in STD rates) will have very different impacts on the transmission of HIV (or any other STD), depending on local prevalence rates and/or the sexual mixing patterns in the population. For this reason, more than any other, it is imperative to evaluate the effectiveness of behavior change interventions by considering the extent to which they change behavior, not merely their impact on the transmission of HIV or other STDs. In addition, although considerably more research is necessary to enable a fuller understanding of the interrelations among behavior change, STD rates, and HIV incidence, a number of models can help determine the impact of a given behavior change in a given population (See Fishbein in http://consensus.nih.gov/1997/1997PreventHIVRisk104PDF.pdf).

Fishbein's account of behavior's influence on HIV infectivity anticipated where we are at this very moment in the history of AIDS. Importantly new tools can manipulate three parameters of the HIV reproductive model. For example, reducing infectiousness, $D$ in the reproductive model, is the premise behind TasP. He also uses the model to explain what we now face with partially effective prevention technologies. What we know about the impact of incomplete condom use in places of lower versus higher HIV prevalence apply just as well to the potential impact of male circumcision in various populations and places. Fishbein introduced the concept of behavioral inoculation, which is central to defining the role of behavior change in combination prevention interventions.

## Evidence Matters

Throughout the 1990s behavioral scientists conducted intervention trials large enough to measure impact on HIV and other STI. Some of these studies faced the challenge of enrolling sufficiently large numbers of people at high risk to analyze reductions in HIV infections. These were expensive studies, costing tens of millions of dollars. Despite the costs and the challenges of conducting prevention trials with biological outcomes, dozens of behavioral intervention trials were undertaken.

Overall HIV risk reduction interventions demonstrate between 25 and 50% increases in condom use—well beyond the 15% that Fishbein showed can impact an HIV epidemic. In an analysis of 11 other meta-analyses, Seth Noar at the University of Kentucky found that every previous review of behavioral prevention trials reported positive increases in condom use, 38% demonstrated reductions in numbers of sex partners and 67% demonstrated significant reductions in STI. Many of the clinical trials that reported positive outcomes were delivered in small group workshops [13]. Groups are cost-efficient and capitalize on social influence to promote and foster behavior change. The largest randomized trial of an HIV prevention intervention delivered to small groups occurred in an NIH sponsored multi-site study called Project Light. In this trial, STI clinic patients were randomized to receive either (a) a 7 group session cognitive and behavioral risk reduction program that focused on condom use, decreasing unprotected sex, and reducing numbers of sex partners or (b) a single 1-h AIDS education group meant to mimic what would typically be offered by community agencies at the time. The results confirmed numerous smaller trials. Condom use increased from 22% of sex acts protected at baseline to 60% during the 1-year follow-up; 43% of the intervention group members reported using condoms consistently every time they had sex, compared to 34% of the comparison group. These behavioral changes were reflected in significant differences in STIs obtained from clinic records. Over the course of 1-year follow-up, for example,

3.6% of men in the risk reduction groups contracted a new case of gonorrhea compared to 6.4% of the comparison group.

Lori Scott-Sheldon of Brown University performed a meta-analysis on behavioral intervention trials aimed at reducing incident STI [14]. The studies were conducted in a variety of high-risk populations in several countries. The analysis included 62 interventions tested in 42 trials that enrolled 40,665 people in North America (62%), Asia (17%), Africa (14%), Europe (5%), and South America (2%). Overall, these behavioral interventions demonstrated significantly fewer incident STI than the control conditions. Importantly, the effects of the behavioral interventions on STI paralleled increased condom use.

In another meta-analysis, Scott-Sheldon and her colleagues evaluated the impact of behavioral interventions that targeted STI clinic patients [15]. This analysis is important because STI clinics are a key point of contact for delivering HIV prevention services. They examined 32 trials that included 67,538 patients in US STI clinics. Results showed that risk reduction counseling and small group workshops reduced sexual risk behaviors over the short term and lowered incident STI in the long term.

One concern with behavioral interventions has been their duration, especially the length and number of sessions. The average small group workshop, for example, has four 90-min sessions. To address this concern behavioral interventionists have worked to shorten interventions. Lisa Eaton at the University of Connecticut conducted another meta-analysis of behavioral interventions aimed to reduce STI, but in this case the interventions were delivered in a single session or "one shot" format. Eaton found that all but 6 of 58 interventions demonstrated significant reductions in incident STI. Overall, single session prevention interventions did surprisingly well, with a 41% reduction in incident STI. Single session interventions are especially important because they can be realistically implemented in clinical settings and could serve as a conduit for delivering TasP.

## Moving the Prevention Goal Posts

In the first decade of AIDS, the challenge posed to behavioral prevention was to demonstrate reductions in unprotected sex and increased condom use. Randomized controlled trials proved this concept with several interventions showing marked reductions in risk behaviors. But the limitations of relying on self-reported sexual behavior created the demand for a second generation of research trials that aimed to demonstrate reductions in STI. As discussed above, several studies tested a wide-variety of interventions that effectively reduce STI. However, HIV transmission is not necessarily the same as other STI. Thus, behavioral interventions were still not embraced as an effective means of HIV prevention.

Stephen Lagakos and Alicia Gable observed the demand for interventions to show effectiveness in preventing HIV infections in their 2008 article "Challenges to HIV Prevention—Seeking Effective Measures in the Absence of a Vaccine" published in the *New England Journal of Medicine* [16]. Lagakos and Gable stated, "Although several behavioral interventions have been shown to reduce self-reported high-risk behaviors and some have reduced the rates of certain non-HIV sexually transmitted infections, none have demonstrated a reduction in the incidence of HIV infection." Carrying a price tag that can exceed $50 million, there are not many intervention trials of the size and scope necessary for testing impact on HIV incidence.

Nancy Padian at the University of California at Berkley systematically reviewed prevention trials aimed to reduce incident HIV infections [17]. She and her colleagues examined the results of 37 studies conducted over 30 years. A total of six randomized trials had significant impacts on HIV infections, five in a preventive direction and one microbicide actually increased HIV transmission. With regard to behavioral interventions designed to reduce HIV infections, they reviewed seven trials, none of which are discussed as effective. The behavioral intervention trials met the same challenges facing many biomedical trials, including poor community engagement, overestimates of HIV incidence, and poor adherence. As Padian and her colleagues discussed, the intervention trials may have been most severely impacted by diminished statistical power resulting from the positive effects of control groups. In fact, when it comes to behavioral interventions, control groups usually share some of the same active ingredients as the experimental interventions.

Nancy Padian's review concluded that prevention interventions aimed to reduce HIV infections reported "flat" results, with no differences between the experimental condition and its control group. In these studies, everyone repeatedly receives HIV testing, counseling, condoms, STI screening, and treatment. It is often the case that both conditions demonstrate reductions in HIV incidence, but not differently from each other. This finding is usually interpreted as a miscalculation of HIV incidence in the cohort, where incidence is lower than originally estimated. Given the effort and resources put into accurately determining HIV incidence in a cohort prior to the trial, repeated miscalculations seem unlikely. An alternative and rarely acknowledged interpretation are the effects of behavioral counseling, testing, screening, etc. that all participants receive. Failure to acknowledge the impact of interventions on STI or even entertain the potential impact of interventions on HIV incidence is perhaps among the most costly oversights in HIV prevention.

## Remembering the MIRA Trial

Based on solid evidence that the cervix and surrounding tissues have high concentrations of cells vulnerable to HIV, Nancy Padian had the idea that protecting the cervix with a contraceptive diaphragm could prevent HIV transmission. The cervix is rich in Langerhans cells, which express receptor sites for HIV attachment and entry. The cervix also has a single layer of cells, whereas other areas of the vagina are better protected with multiple cell layers. There is also evidence that the diaphragm is effective in protecting women from other STI, including gonorrhea. The biological plausibility that the diaphragm could prevent HIV transmission is therefore quite compelling. Unlike the female condom, the diaphragm is truly female controlled, inexpensive, and widely available. The case was convincing and the diaphragm was tested for HIV prevention in the MIRA Trial, one of the more carefully planned intervention trials in HIV prevention history.

A total of 5,045 women in southern Africa participated in MIRA [18]. All women in the study received intensive HIV testing and risk reduction counseling every 6 months. Women in the experimental condition were fitted and trained in proper use of the diaphragm. For ethical reasons, women were told that the only known method of preventing HIV infection during sex is with male condoms. As described by Padian and her colleagues in the MIRA project intervention protocol (MIRA Trial Standard Operating Procedure, 2005):

> At each visit, women received a 3-month supply of gel, and were counseled that the effectiveness of the diaphragm and lubricant gel for the prevention of HIV infection was not known. To prevent HIV, they were asked to use condoms regardless of whether or not they used the diaphragm and lubricant gel. Participants were also told that they should not use the diaphragm and lubricant alone as a method of contraception. The diaphragm is approved for contraception when used with a spermicide (typical effectiveness 84%), but its effectiveness without nonoxynol-9 has not been fully established

The content of the safer sex counseling that all participants received throughout the study is also described in the study protocol as:

> Safer Sex and Condom Use Counseling will be provided at screening, enrollment and at every follow-up visit. Correct-Use Demonstrations will be done by counselors at screening and enrollment and offered at every follow-up visit. Women should also be offered the opportunity to practice condom insertion on the penis model at every visit. If the participant declines a demonstration or practice at a follow-up visit, the counselor should ensure that this is because the woman is comfortable with the procedures and provide chart notes. The counselor at each site will use a standardized script to provide each study participant with information on methods of HIV transmission, prevention and safe sex (including the proper use of condoms). Counseling about using the condoms as a study product should be provided to all participants at each follow-up visit. Participants in the diaphragm and gel arm should always be reminded that it is not yet proven that these products protect against HIV or STI, and that therefore, it is advisable always to use male condoms. The use of male condoms with all partners, including primary and non-primary partners, should be emphasized for protection against HIV and STIs. Due to the possibility of creating friction that might make women vulnerable to HIV/STIs, participants are not advised to use female condoms while the diaphragm is inserted.

A "safer sex counseling script" was included in the counseling protocol that included the following behavioral recommendations:

- Ensure a confidential environment
- Explain that latex condoms provide the best protection from many STIs, including HIV
- Encourage the participant to use condoms with every act of sexual intercourse regardless or whether she feels at risk for HIV/STIs
- Explain the importance of discussing condom use with partner(s)

- Identify any difficulties the participant perceives
- Assist the participant in building skills to negotiate condom use with partner(s) through discussion and role-plays, as needed
- Discuss potential problems with condoms, including breakage and slippage
- Discuss proper storage of condoms, and from where she is getting her condoms
- Discourage use of any vaginal products including douche, traditional substances such as herbs, or other lubricants
- Discourage use of any spermicides, including any products containing non-oxynol-9 such as spermicidal-lubricated condoms
- Using the penis model, show the participant how to put a condom on and take it off (Required at screening and enrollment and must be offered at follow-up)
- Offer the participant the opportunity to practice putting a condom on the penis model

Women who were randomly assigned to the experimental group also received a fitted diaphragm, with instructions for proper use with Replens, a lubricating gel with antimicrobial properties. The study was designed to detect a 33% reduction in HIV incidence between women who received the diaphragm and women who did not.

Overall, the results of MIRA showed no differences between the groups in reducing HIV incidence. That is, just as many women who received the diaphragm became infected with HIV as women who did not. Women in both study conditions significantly reduced their unprotected sexual exposure to HIV; more than 90% of women in both groups used a barrier the last time they had sex. Women in the control group demonstrated a high rate of condoms, offering 90% protection against HIV. In contrast, 53% of women who received the diaphragm used condoms the last time they had sex, whereas 37% used the diaphragm. Although women were instructed to use both the diaphragm and condom, the lower condom use in the intervention group shows that women substituted a product with unknown protective value, the diaphragm, for condoms with known protection. Women who were most likely to substitute using the diaphragm in place of condoms were the same women who most believed the diaphragm would protect them against HIV. This pattern of results is similar to that seen in studies of female condoms, where efforts to increase female condoms result in greater use of both male and female condoms. The motivations and skills for using one barrier method probably generalize to use other barriers as well.

The MIRA Trial is generally discussed as a failure to demonstrate the diaphragm as an effective means of preventing HIV transmission. The rules of interpreting this carefully conducted randomized clinical trial dictate this strict interpretation. However, the findings seem to tell us much more. First, the study should be considered a massively successful demonstration of HIV testing and counseling for sustained protection against HIV infection. Repeated testing and risk reduction counseling led to condom use with 90% protection at last intercourse in the control group.

HIV incidence in the MIRA Trial was lower than estimated at the start. Incidence may have gone down for any number of reasons outside of the interventions delivered, so we cannot definitively conclude the counseling and testing resulted in the reduction. Given that HIV incidence among women in southern Africa was not declining or even stable, delivering semiannual HIV testing and counseling to women and encouraging condom use every 6 months surely must be considered a likely contributor to the reduced HIV incidence. Second, the study findings suggest that the diaphragm is as effective as condoms at preventing HIV infections. Women who received the diaphragm were half as likely to use condoms the last time they had sex, and yet they were no more likely to become infected. If you believe the data, it is reasonable to conclude that the comparable protection observed in the two groups could only result if the diaphragm was effective in preventing HIV infection. This interpretation is consistent with the declining rate of HIV incidence in the cohort. Still, we must conclude that the diaphragm was not shown effective because it did not surpass the impact of repeat testing, counseling, and condom access. However, a common sense approach to the data suggests that this biologically plausible device worked at least as well as condoms in preventing HIV infection.

## Remembering Project Explore

The need to determine whether an intensive behavioral intervention can reduce HIV infections was answered by Project Explore multicenter trial led by Beryl Koblin of the New York Blood Center [19]. Project Explore enrolled 4,295 men who have sex with men between 1999 and 2003 in six US cities—Boston, Chicago, Denver, New York, San Francisco, and Seattle. The intervention was developed by Margaret Chesney at the University of California at San Francisco and represented the best of what we know about HIV prevention. The counseling was based on principles of motivational interviewing and social-cognitive behavioral skills building models for health behavior change [20]. Chesney conducted preliminary work to identify key behavioral targets. For example, 75% of gay men had reported sexual pleasure as the central basis for engaging in unprotected anal sex, forming the basis for motivational interviewing. Substance use was also a prominent feature of risk among men in the formative research and therefore became a major focus of the counseling. Men randomized to the Explore intervention received ten prevention modules in just as many sessions over 4–6 months. Each session lasted an average of just under 40 min. Table 1.2 displays the core components of the ten counseling modules. In the end, nearly 75% of Explore participants had received all of the sessions, with an additional 12% receiving between six and nine sessions. Men who received Explore counseling were also provided with maintenance counseling every 3 months, as well as HIV testing every 6 months for the duration of the study. Men in the comparison intervention received HIV testing every 6 months accompanied by counseling that has been shown to reduce STI [21].

**Table 1.2** Counseling modules, core themes, and session descriptions from project explore (adapted from [20])

| Module | Core theme | Session focus |
|---|---|---|
| Module 1 | Being HIV negative and participating in EXPLORE | Participants state why they want to stay HIV negative; desire to remain negative is made explicit<br>Mixed feelings about sex and risk are examined and normalized, beginning the focus on ambivalence |
| Modules 2 and 3 | Risk: What's acceptable to me?<br>Crossing acceptable risk limits | Knowledge of risk factors for infection is assessed<br>Personal relevance of risk reduction guidelines is examined through recent sexual episode narratives; individual attitudes regarding "acceptable" risk<br>Discussion regarding pleasure of unprotected sex |
| Modules 4 and 5 | Sexual communication: HIV status, spoken and unspoken messages | Attitudes and skills that facilitate or impair clear communication of risk limits; communication about serostatus; the role of being part of a couple that employs risk limits or negotiated safety arrangements |
| Module 6 | Sex, drinking, and drugs | Impact of substance use on risk behavior |
| Modules 7, 8, and 9 | Places and events as triggers<br>Feelings and thoughts as triggers<br>Partners as triggers | How personal, social, and environmental factors may trigger risky sex or preventative behavior<br>Examination and skills training to manage risk when presented with<br>• Places where risky sex may occur<br>• Life and social events that may encourage risk<br>• Emotions and self-talk that cue risk taking<br>• Partner characteristics that trigger risky sex |
| Module 10 | Planning for maintenance<br>Staying HIV negative | Planning for ongoing adherence to personal safety plans, including training for relapse prevention; applying lessons from modules to changing life situations |

The Project Explore Trial was designed to test reductions in HIV incidence. In Project Explore, effectiveness was defined at the outset as reducing HIV incidence by 35%. The decision rules are stated in study protocol and final outcome paper. As stated in the Explore Trial Executive Summary:

> To be specific, the EXPLORE study was designed so that the intervention strategy would be declared beneficial if the reduction in HIV incidence was statistically significantly above 10% (that is, that the lower bound of the confidence interval was above 10%). If not, and the reduction in HIV incidence was statistically significantly below 35% (that is, the upper bound of the confidence interval was below 35%), the benefit of the intervention strategy would be ruled out. In case neither was true, the intervention would be considered plausibly efficacious with merit for further evaluation, possibly with select refinements. With the target sample size of 4,350 and an expected HIV incidence of 1.55 per 100 person-years in the standard arm, if the true reduction in HIV incidence was 35%, there would be 3.0% chance of ruling out benefit, 50.0% chance of declaring benefit, and 46.9% chance of stating plausibly efficacious. Furthermore, if the true reduction in HIV incidence was 0%, there would be an 75.0% chance of ruling out benefit (Explore Executive Summary [22], p. 3).

Thus, the researchers stated from the start that if the intervention did not reduce HIV incidence by 35% it would be deemed ineffective. As it turned out, the Explore counseling did reduce HIV incidence by 39% the first year after counseling. However, the difference in incidence between the Explore Counseling and its control group reduced to 18.2% by the 48-month follow-up. Thus, not effective, but promising. Although I have been unable to locate a reference for defining success as a 35% reduction in HIV incidence, this benchmark seems grounded in the same epidemiological principles that are set forth in vaccine trials. Unlike vaccines, however, the lifelong protection offered by risk reduction counseling and other adherence dependent interventions couldn't realistically be expected. The implications of declaring Project Explore ineffective are profound because nearly 30 years of behavioral intervention research is mistakenly discarded. With the exception of an effective vaccine, which we do not have, and male circumcision, all HIV prevention technologies require long-term behavior change and sustained adherence. Trials that are stopped early because they show immediate compelling evidence for efficacy may not be efficacious 48 months later. This point will become important when we consider the definitive evidence for the efficacy of TasP. At least with behavioral counseling we know what to expect given that Project Explore was not stopped early.

The basis for the study sample size was derived from previous vaccine preparedness studies (VPS). Cohorts of high-risk populations were enrolled, tested, and counseled over time as they waited for a vaccine trial to commence. Vaccine preparedness studies that enrolled men who have sex with men in the USA demonstrated overall incidence of new HIV infections that averaged 1.55 infections per 100 person-years. Based on observations in the vaccine preparedness cohorts, it was determined prior to the start of the study that a difference between the conditions of less than 35% in HIV incidence would be considered non-substantial.

Although incidence rates vary over time, most estimates of HIV incidence for men who have sex with men seemed stable, typically ranging between 1.2 and 1.8 HIV

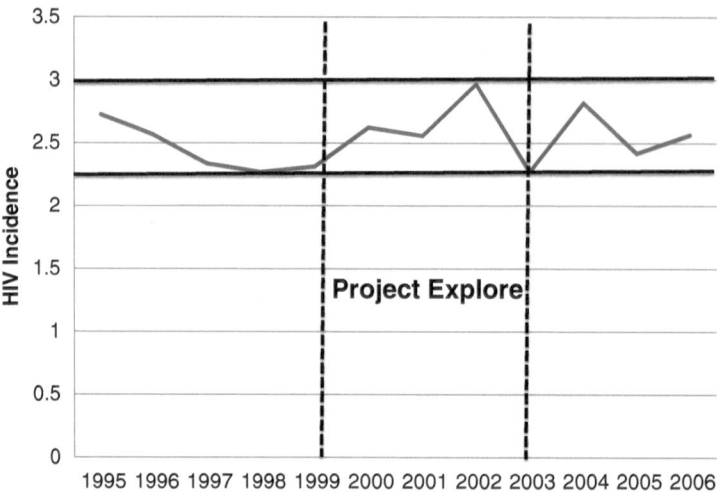

**Fig. 1.1** Estimated HIV incidence in US cities during the years before, during, and after Project Explore, 1995–2006 (Data from Stall et al. [23] used with permission)

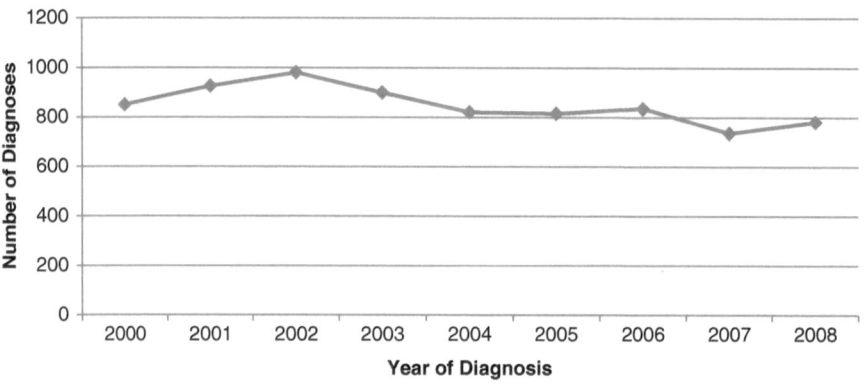

**Fig. 1.2** Rates of HIV infections in Chicago, 2000–2008 (*Source*: City of Chicago Department of Health)

infections per 100 person-years. In a review of HIV incidence among MSM, Ron Stall at the University of Pittsburgh has shown that incidence has remained mostly stable over the HIV epidemic; 2.39 HIV infections per 100 person-years in community samples, 2.45 in alternative HIV testing sites, and 3.84 among men receiving care at STI clinics [23]. Overall, men who have sex with men in North America demonstrate an HIV incidence of 2.6 per 100 persons years. As shown in Fig. 1.1, the HIV incidence rates reported by Ron Stall as well as in cities that participated in Project Explore showed very little change between 1999 and 2003, the years that Project Explore was conducted. Similar stable patterns are seen in the cities where Explore was conducted, such as Chicago (see Fig. 1.2). Furthermore, data from behavioral

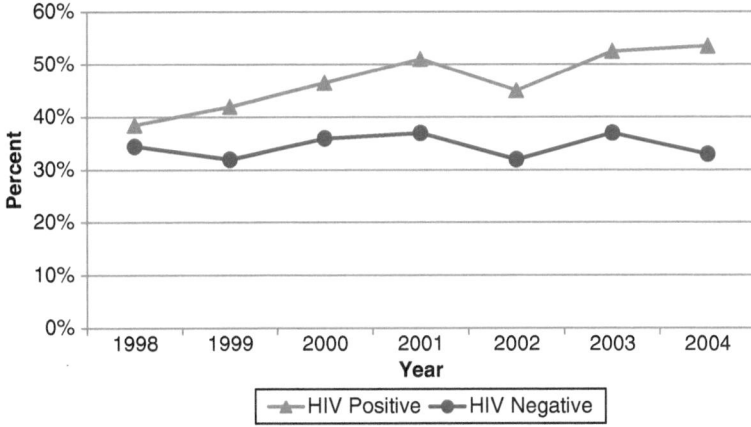

**Fig. 1.3** Percent of MSM reporting unprotected anal intercourse by self-reported HIV status in San Francisco, 1998–2004 (*Source*: City of San Francisco Department of Health)

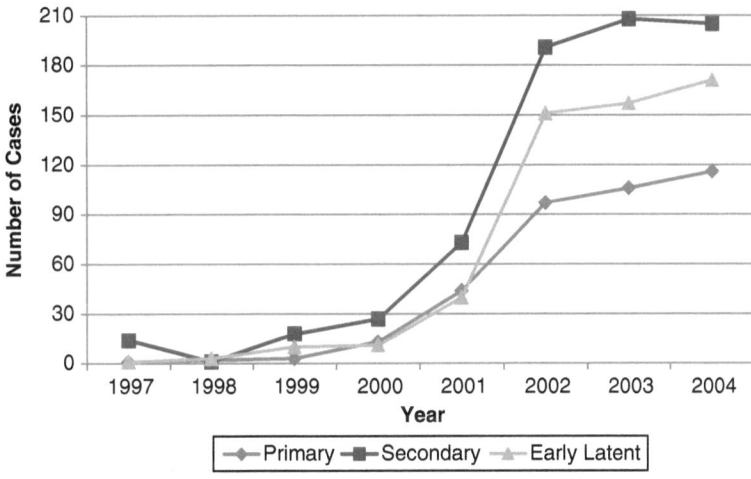

**Fig. 1.4** Number of primary, secondary, and tertiary Syphilis cases among MSM in San Francisco, 1997–2004 (*Source*: City of San Francisco Department of Health)

and STI surveillance in San Francisco shows increases in MSM unprotected anal sex and STI during the years of Project Explore (see Figs. 1.3 and 1.4).

In Project Explore, the counseling and control conditions both demonstrated reductions in high-risk behaviors, with the Explore counseling reducing unprotected anal intercourse by a factor of 20.5% greater than the control group. The HIV incidence outcomes are shown in Figs. 1.5 and 1.6. Over 48 months of follow-up, the HIV incidence for men who received the Explore counseling was 1.9 infections per

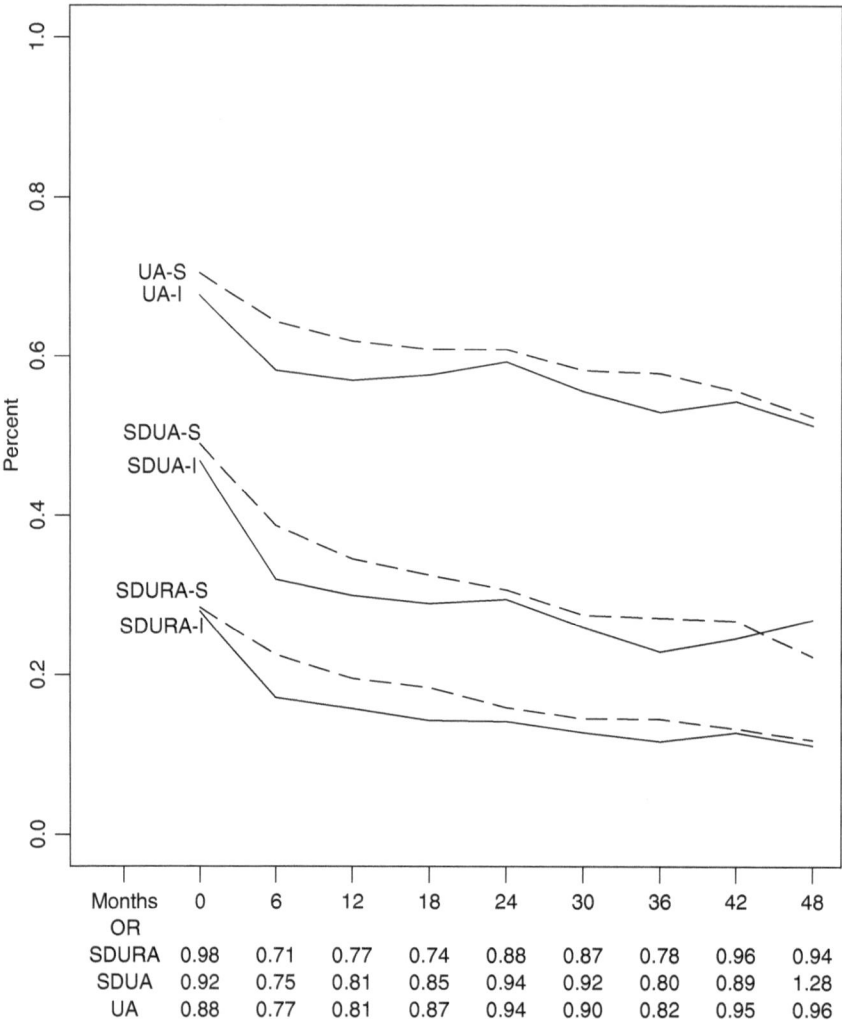

**Fig. 1.5** Percent engaging in sexual risk behavior outcomes over 48 months follow-up from the Project Explore intervention trial. *UA-S* unprotected anal sex for standard condition, *UA-I* unprotected anal sex for intervention condition, *SDUA-S* serodiscordant unprotected anal sex for standard condition, *SDUA-I* serodiscordant unprotected anal sex for intervention condition, *SDURA-S* serodiscordant unprotected receptive anal sex for standard condition, *SDURA-I* serodiscordant unprotected receptive anal sex for intervention condition, *OR* odds ratio (Koblin et al. [19] used with permission)

100 person-years, compared to 2.3 per 100,000 for men who received semiannual testing and counseling, an 18% difference. Thus, over the course of 4 years (average follow-up 3.25 years), the difference between the conditions was not considered significant. However, the shorter-term outcomes of Explore counseling did clear the 35% difference in HIV incidence.

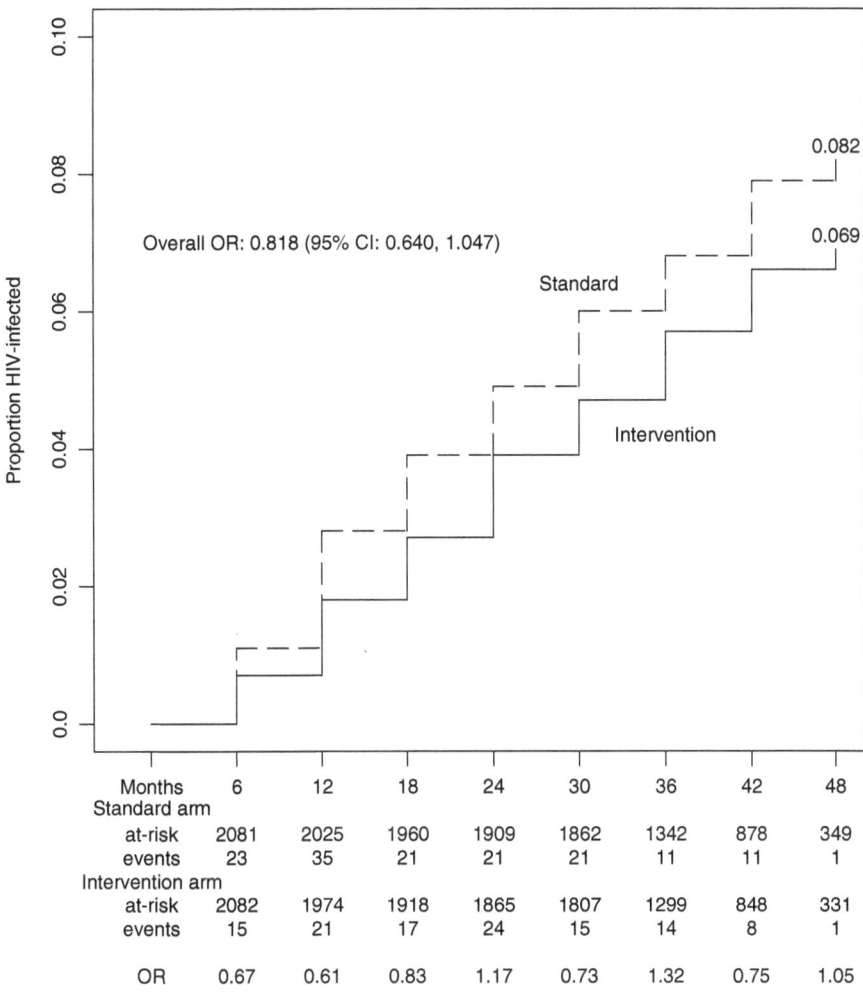

**Fig. 1.6** Proportion HIV incidence outcomes for standard and intervention conditions from the Project Explore intervention trial (Koblin et al. [19] used with permission)

In 2008 Tom Coates of the University of California at Los Angeles, one of the lead Explore investigators, stated that "The effects of the intervention on HIV incidence seemed to be substantial in the first 12 months, with a 33% reduction in the first 6 months and a 39% reduction in the first 12 months. But the intervention and control groups did not differ significantly in HIV incidence at the end of the 3.25 years of follow-up. Had the study terminated when behavioral studies are usually stopped (i.e., at 12-months' follow-up), the intervention would have been declared effective."

Concluding that Project Explore did not demonstrate significant reductions in HIV incidence seems absurd. No other HIV prevention intervention of any kind has been held to a 3-year standard for long-term outcomes. In addition, only those participants enrolled in the first year of the study, a fairly small number of men to reliably assess HIV incidence, could be represented in the long-term outcomes. It seems implausible that the reductions in HIV incidence can be accounted for by anything other than the behavioral interventions delivered in both trial conditions. Whether policy makers accept the results of Project Explore as demonstrating that behavioral interventions can avert HIV infections, or rather dismiss them as promising, may determine whether behavioral counseling will be integrated with TasP.

## Behavioral Interventions to Enhance Treatment Adherence

Behavioral interventions to enhance HIV treatment adherence have proven successful in helping patients adhere to their medications and ultimately suppress viral replication. Effective adherence interventions have drawn from the same theories of behavior change as HIV prevention interventions. Meta-analyses of controlled interventions demonstrate positive outcomes, with impacts on increased adherence and reductions in HIV viral load. Rivet Amico of the University of Connecticut, for example, has shown that behavioral interventions to improve treatment adherence consistently result in clinically meaningful improvements in adherence [24]. Jane Simoni at the University of Washington reports similarly impressive results [25, 26]. Relatively brief behavioral interventions tested in randomized controlled trials often yield greater than 90% medication adherence, with similar effects in achieving undetectable viral loads. Improved adherence resulting from behavioral interventions can even exceed improvements observed from simplified medication regimens. For example, Jean-Jacques Parienti of the Université Pierre et Marie Curie in Paris studied the impact of once-daily antiretroviral therapy regimens on adherence and found a significant but small improvement over twice-daily regimens. Thus, behavioral interventions will play a critical role in facilitating adherence in TasP [27].

Colleen DiIorio at Emory University tested one adherence intervention of particular relevance to TasP [28, 29]. This intervention used a motivational interviewing framework to assist people in understanding their medications and how they work to suppress HIV, learn the importance of adherence and develop strategies for maintaining medication adherence. Patients rated their motivation and confidence for adhering to their medication regimen, the counseling explored ways to further improve their adherence, and patients entered into an adherence contract with their counselor. DiIorio and her colleagues found significant improvements in medication adherence with twice as many patients in the control condition reporting missing medications during the follow-up period than those who received counseling.

Further evidence in support of DiIorio's adherence intervention comes from a meta-analysis and content evaluation of adherence interventions with standard of care control groups. Marijn de Bruin at Waleningen University in the Netherlands created an index for the number of behavior change techniques or strategies that people in the experimental conditions received [30]. Interventions that delivered the greatest number of behavioral adherence strategies demonstrated the greatest proportion of persons attaining high levels of adherence and undetectable viral loads. DiIorio's brief motivational interviewing adherence intervention discussed above demonstrated considerable capacity, meaning that patients received multiple behavioral strategies and demonstrated substantial improvements in adherence. The brief motivational counseling also occurred in a clinical context, supporting its feasibility and ecological validity. The strong standard of care surely contributed to the overall impact of the counseling, but the randomized design provides evidence that the motivational counseling added value above and beyond usual clinical services. The conceptual basis for DiIorio's adherence counseling matches the conceptual basis for effective risk reduction counseling, suggesting the two may easily be melded together. Brief motivational counseling is highly adaptive and offers an excellent vehicle for delivering behavioral counseling in the context of TasP.

Stand-alone adherence interventions are already delivered in routine clinical care. Rivet Amico conducted a survey of clinicians who care for HIV/AIDS patients and found that most providers deliver routine adherence counseling which often encompasses the same components as found in state of the science interventions. For example, 78% of providers deliver individual adherence counseling, 58% conduct supportive adherence groups, and 47% use pre-prescription training groups to bolster adherence [31]. Providers also utilize many of the behavioral strategies and adherence devices shown effective in intervention trials; 88% provide patients with pillboxes and medication organizers, 41% use instructional brochures and handouts, and 35% have patients keep medication journals or calendars. These same providers will likely become the frontline implementers of TasP. It is only a slight pivot from the current standard of care to new models built on motivational counseling that can integrate adherence with risk reduction strategies.

## Behavioral Principles for TasP

The future of HIV prevention does not rest on any particular behavioral intervention model or prevention package or even theory of behavior change. One of the great myths in HIV prevention has been that effective interventions have unique formulae that must be followed with fidelity for positive results. The marketing of prevention interventions has propagated this myth as products delivered in a box, with a manual, fixed procedures, and copyrighted materials. The "programs in a box" approach has paid more attention to the surface or appearance of intervention activities than to their underlying mechanisms and principles. A successful implementation of TaSP will demand an agile approach to behavioral principles that can be adapted and blended with treatments for delivery in broad contexts and to an array of populations.

Mary Jane Rotheram-Borus is at the forefront of distilling effective interventions to their basic foundations. She and her colleagues at the University of California at Los Angeles examined five different interventions designed to reduce HIV risk behaviors in adolescents. The interventions were tested and found effective in carefully conducted clinical trials. Each intervention is included in the CDC's dissemination of effective interventions. Rotheram-Borus identified principles, factors, and processes shared across all of the interventions. She defines principles as program content themes or the stated goals and anticipated lessons learned from an intervention activity [32]. The ten common principles of effective HIV prevention are:

- Believe in your own worth and your right to a happy future
- Distinguish fact from myth
- Evaluate options and consequences
- Commit to change
- Plan ahead and be prepared
- Practice self-control
- Know pleasurable alternatives to high-risk sexual activity
- Negotiate verbally, not nonverbally
- Choose to limit your own freedom
- Act to help others protect themselves

Rotheram-Borus has gone a step further to identify common factors that cut across effective risk reduction interventions. Common factors are conceptualized at the highest level of abstraction; structural features of effective programs from which content and processes are drawn. Common factors move us away from any one theory, activity, or curriculum. Rotheram-Borus argues that effective behavioral interventions may appear different, but they obtain very similar outcomes because they derive their content from shared common factors [33]. She identified five common factors of effective HIV prevention interventions:

- Establish a framework to understand behavior change
- Convey issue-specific and population-specific information
- Build cognitive, affective, and behavioral self-management skills
- Address environmental barriers to implementing health behaviors
- Provide tools to develop ongoing social and community support

Finally, Rotheram-Borus describes common change processes of effective interventions. She and her colleagues differentiate change processes from intervention processes, which are generally considered treatment techniques or delivery devices [34]. They identified 19 common processes categorized as three structural features:

- Group management strategies
- Competence building
- Addressing developmental challenges

They found that all effective programs, at least for adolescents, shared the same structural features (e.g., goal setting and session agendas), used an active engagement style of group management, and built cognitive competence.

Effective behavioral approaches to TasP will share these same common principles, factors, and processes. Building on these foundations for effective implementation of TasP will also encompass unique features. The following are a few such areas for expansion of behavioral principles to meet the challenges and opportunities of TasP.

## Effectively Communicate Partial Protection

With the exception of abstinence, 100% condom use, and clean needles, no approach to HIV prevention is likely to exceed 80% protection against HIV. Even with perfect adherence, TasP does not render people noninfectious. Thus, at its best TasP must be considered partially protective. Unfortunately, partial protection is not so easy to communicate. The concept is more meaningful for forecasting prevention impacts on epidemiologic trends than it is for communicating personal risk. Mathematical models may find that a 35% reduction in HIV incidence is sufficient to reduce HIV in a population, but what does that mean to an individual? If a man is told that his HIV positive male sex partner has an undetectable viral load it will reduce his risk for HIV by 90%, assuming his partner takes his medication and does not have an STI, how should he interpret this information? Should he still use condoms? Can he use condoms less? Does 90% protection mean he should only use condoms one in ten times he has sex? And what if his partner misses taking his medications? What if his partner has genital herpes? These are very real questions that do not yet have answers.

TasP counseling should explain partial protection and appraise the individual's acceptance of lower, but not eliminated, risks. Decisional balance exercises, for example, help individuals weigh their risks and make informed decisions about which of several options may suite them best. Understanding partial protection also means dispelling myths and correcting misperceptions. People generally want to feel safe. However, false safety beliefs actually increase risk. Partially protective prevention technologies require that people understand their risks and how treatments may reduce, but not eliminate, their risks. Motivating people to adhere to treatment when the primary purpose is prevention will undoubtedly be a key to success.

## Reduce Risk Compensation

Risk compensation is a well-known cognitive-behavioral phenomenon that may very well be the Achilles Heel of TasP [35]. Risk compensation should not, however, be confused with behavioral disinhibition. Unlike behavioral disinhibition, risk compensation is based on an internalized risk calculus, where behavior is adjusted in response to changes in risk producing circumstances. It occurs when people feel safer after taking protective action and adjust their behavior to maintain their "accepted level" of risk. For example, people drive faster when they have anti-lock brakes or when they wear seat belts. Research shows that bicyclists have lower risk perceptions and ride with greater risk when wearing a protective helmet. For example, Ross Phillips and his colleagues reported an experiment that showed bike riders who typically wear helmets increased cycling speed and decreased their risk perceptions when wearing helmets compared to when they were not wearing helmets [36]. According to Risk Homeostasis Theory, decreases in perceived risk occur with access to prevention technologies and correspond with increases in risk behavior. Knowing how individuals perceive their risk for HIV is a critical step in estimating the ultimate impact of TasP. People who engage in risk behaviors accept a certain level of risk. The idea is that risk behaviors are balanced against risk perceptions and perceived benefits that accompany behavioral adjustments. As circumstances change, such as the availability of risk reducing technologies, estimates of personal risk are altered and behaviors are adjusted.

The first step in maintaining risk homeostasis is to determine the level of risk a person is willing to accept. Because contracting HIV is such a devastating health risk, the threshold of acceptable risk is pretty low. Determining a target set point for risk generally involves some internal analysis of the costs and benefits of the relative protective and risk behaviors. Once a person sets a target set point they engage in a comparative process between perceived risks and target levels of risk they are willing to take. A person who believes that because their risk for HIV is cut in half when their sex partner is being treated for HIV will likely use condoms less. In vaccine preparedness studies, believing that a vaccine is protective may increase risk behavior by as much as 50% [37, 38]. Mathematical models that estimate the overall impact of TasP show that even modest increases in numbers of partners or unprotected sex could offset preventive benefits [39].

Risk compensation clearly occurred in the South African male circumcision trial, and seemed to occur in the circumcision trial conducted in Kenya [40–43]. It is probably impossible to observe risk compensation in a randomized prevention trial because people are constantly monitored and counseled. Risk compensation is a real-world phenomenon that requires real-world approaches to research.

## Maintain Adherence

All prevention approaches except male circumcision or perhaps a vaccine are adherence dependent. The antiretroviral-based microbicide gel tested in the CAPRISA 004 trial demonstrated 54% reduction in risk for women who used the product more than 80% of the time, as compared to 28% protection for women who used the gel less than 50% [44]. Previously tested microbicides may have failed to demonstrate efficacy because of poor adherence. For example, the Carraguard microbicide was used on average 44% of the time and only 10% of women stated that they always used the gel before sex [6]. Even if Carraguard had worked it would have failed for incomplete adherers. Similarly, men who have sex with men who received antiretroviral preexposure prevention (PrEP) in the iPrEx trial demonstrated 44% protection against HIV, with the highest degree of protection occurring among men with the greatest drug concentrations in their blood [45]. Antiretroviral-based prevention strategies demonstrate dose–response relationships much the same as therapeutic uses of these same drugs. We should therefore not expect suboptimal adherence to treatment to work any better for TasP than it does for disease management.

## Briefer Can Be Better

Another myth in HIV prevention is that longer duration interventions will have greater impact on behavior change. Some of the first behavior change interventions required as many as 12 small group sessions. Although multiple small group sessions worked well in research settings, asking people to come to these interventions proved infeasible. It also became apparent that much of the time spent in the sessions was extraneous, often focused on rapport building and delivering information, neither of which have shown much impact on behavior.

In response to the limitations of multiple session prevention programs, single session or "one shot" interventions have become a focus of research. Brief workshops as well as single session risk reduction counseling have proven to be just as effective as their much longer, more demanding, and expensive multisession counterparts. The greater efficiency of single session prevention interventions should have great appeal for use with TasP. The same is true for medication adherence interventions, where relatively brief models have proven effective as well as efficient.

Briefer behavioral interventions cost less and therefore offer a greater public health value. The new era of prevention places a premium on efficiency as well as efficacy. Shorter interventions will ultimately be the most useful. Take for example client-centered risk reduction counseling delivered with HIV testing. As the CDC has demonstrated, counseling can be delivered in only 20 min with significant long-term impacts on STI.

But despite our best efforts to simultaneously condense and intensify interventions, clinical service providers often complain that even 20-min risk reduction interventions are infeasible in public health practice. For this reason, the CDC no longer requires client-centered counseling in combination with HIV testing. If current health services are too burdened and under-resourced to accommodate even a single 20-min counseling session, the outlook for TasP is bleak. Without creative structural changes to the health care system, TasP will in all likelihood be doomed to merely dispensing prescription refills.

## Bridge the Digital Divide

The costs and resource demands of behavioral interventions are also reduced by smart technologies. At the most basic level, video has proven quite effective in delivering information, role model stories, and risk scenarios. Lance Weinhardt conducted research with STI clinic patients and found great interest in computer-delivered interventions. Patients at a large urban clinic indicated that they saw several advantages to computerized prevention programs including the impartiality of advice given by a computerized counselor, privacy or confidentiality, accuracy of information, convenience, and the ability to control the flow of information. Weinhardt and his colleagues constructed a computerized intervention designed to augment risk reduction counseling. The intervention proved efficient and feasible in a busy clinical setting [46].

Behavioral interventions have also been completely computerized for use in clinic settings. Although not every approach has worked, there are important advances in computerized interventions. Diane Grimley at the University of Alabama tested a 15-min risk reduction intervention for use in STI clinics [47]. The intervention was based on the Stages of Health Behavior Change Model and was designed to move clients through a self-assessment, risk awareness, and stage-tailored steps of risk reduction. A randomized clinical trial compared the computerized intervention to a control group that only completed a computerized multiple health risk assessment. The results showed that in addition to increased condom use, 6% of participants who received the brief computerized counseling intervention were diagnosed with chlamydia and/or gonorrhea at the 6-month follow-up, compared to 13% of the control group, more than a 50% difference in risk reduction. When Grimley compared the intervention effects with baseline STI prevalence, the risk reduction program decreased STI by 22% compared to a 3% reduction in the comparison group [48]. Grimley concluded "that a single, interactive, computer-delivered intervention at the evaluation visit can increase consistent condom use and reduce STDs without putting any additional burden on clinic staff."

Promising effects have also emerged from completely computerized interventions to enhance HIV treatment adherence. Jeff Fisher and his colleagues tested a computerized program to improve medication adherence developed for use in infectious disease clinic waiting rooms [49]. The program consists of several components that included a tutorial, introduction to a virtual guide who accompanies patients through the intervention experience, assessments, goal setting, and 20 adherence promotion activities. The first session focused on developing adherence promotion strategies that address adherence barriers and choosing an adherence-related goal. The average time spent to complete a full intervention visit was 26 min with an average of 8 min devoted specifically to adherence. Subsequent sessions occurred at regularly scheduled clinic appointments as patients waited to see their provider. "Check-in" sessions were patient-linked and focused on goal progress as well as additional intervention activities. The results showed that patients who received the intervention were significantly more likely to achieve 100% self-reported adherence compared to those who only received usual care. Although the effects on viral suppression were not statistically significant, the reported trends suggest some clinical benefit from the intervention.

Cell phone and smart phone technologies can also play a key role in advancing TasP. Nancy Reynolds of Yale University developed and tested a telephone delivered adherence intervention based on Self-Regulation Theory [50]. This model emphasized skills and strategies for health monitoring, cognitive appraisal, stress management, and behavioral control. The intervention demonstrated significant improvements in medication adherence and viral suppression. My research group adapted Reynold's model for delivery in four brief biweekly cell phone delivered counseling sessions. Our intervention used unannounced phone-based pill counts for medication monitoring with problem solving and medication management coaching sessions. In an initial pilot test of the behavioral self-regulation counseling intervention, we found that participants who received self-management counseling demonstrated improved adherence immediately after the final session and 1 month after counseling.

New and emerging technologies for improving medication adherence will also play important roles in TasP. Jessica Haberer of Harvard University has found that an electronic pillbox that uses cellular technology called "Wise-pill" can be used in urban and rural settings in developed and developing countries. Dose-linked behavior is monitored in real time by communicating date-time stamped container openings. Failure to receive a signal at the clinic means the container was not opened, allowing the provider to intervene. Wise-pill and other electronic devices are revolutionizing behavioral interventions for medication adherence, with direct relevance to TasP.

## Seize (or Create) Teachable Moments

Timing may be the single most important predictor of intervention success. Brief interventions are particularly dependent on teachable moments as they offer a window of opportunity for behavior change. Teachable moments can occur during periods of heightened risk awareness. That is, individuals are more open to change when experiencing a sense of personal vulnerability. There are numerous examples of how teachable moments can facilitate health behavior change. For example, sudden commitments to change can occur in smokers who experience chest pain, alcoholics with elevated liver enzymes, obese persons who are diagnosed borderline diabetic, and individuals diagnosed with an STI [51]. Circumstances that are most promising for creating teachable moments are those experienced as a "close call," or when a person feels they have "dodged a bullet."

McBride and colleagues [52, 53] described three features that define teachable moments:

- Increases in personal perceptions of risk and altered outcome expectancies
- Prompting strong emotional responses
- Redefines self-concept and social roles

HIV testing results, condom breaks, partner infidelities, learning a partner has HIV, and contracting an STI can enhance a sense of personal vulnerability to HIV. These experiences also evoke strong emotional responses like threat, anger, and betrayal that can redefine relationships and roles.

Teachable moments seem especially critical for brief interventions, which require attention and motivation. And yet, it will not always be the case that interventions are poised in the midst of a teachable moment. Researchers are therefore developing techniques to create teachable moments within the context of prevention interventions. Lisa Eaton, for example, developed an activity used in risk reduction counseling to create a teachable moment. Her intervention is a 40-min risk reduction counseling session designed for HIV negative men who have sex with men who serosort—that is select sex partners based on their perceived HIV negative status. At the start of the counseling session clients read a graphic novel-style story of a man named Mike, who only practices unprotected anal sex with men who tell him that they are also HIV negative. Mike believes he is safe, but he gets tested regularly just to be sure. The story ends with Mike in shock when he receives a positive HIV test result. The story of Mike is intended to heighten awareness, effectively creating a teachable moment after which the counselor picks up where the story leaves off. The discussion leads to a personalized sexual network activity that explores partners and risk perceptions, followed by risk reduction strategies. It is easy to imagine a similar approach to creating teachable moments to set the stage for TasP counseling.

## Wanted: A Theoretical Framework for TasP

The current state of HIV prevention demands creative behavioral strategies used in combination with antiretroviral therapies. Behavioral theories of the past have relied on cognitive, rational, and reasoned explanations for sexual and drug use practices. Behavioral theories have become an alphabet soup of psychological constructs. These models served the field for nearly 30 years and yielded numerous evidence-based prevention interventions. Still, the theories themselves fall short and do not get to the heart of what are essentially physiological, emotional, intimate, and power-based behaviors. It seems the best models have been able to achieve is to emphasize motivation, but even then motivation is reduced to intentions, goals, attitudes, and other cognitive constructs. What we need are theories to account for sexual and addictive behaviors that can translate to combinations of evidence-based interventions.

UNAIDS defines combination HIV prevention as "The strategic, simultaneous use of different classes of prevention activities (biomedical, behavioral, community, societal) that operate on multiple levels (individual, relationship, social/structural), to respond to the needs of particular audiences and modes of HIV transmission, and to make efficient use of resources through prioritizing, partnership, and engagement of affected communities" [54]. Drawing a direct parallel to highly active antiretroviral therapy itself, King Holmes of the University of Washington was among the first to articulate the concept of highly active HIV prevention. Any single antiretroviral medication will only partially suppress HIV replication, and quickly results in resistance. King Holmes sees HIV prevention interventions operating in the same way; all are partially effective and of limited use by themselves. Tom Coates moved the concept of highly active HIV prevention forward by discussing the synergism of prevention strategies [55]. The combined effects of additional approaches strengthen each individual strategy.

Roger Tatoud of Imperial College in London states that the pace of new HIV infections drives the need for new HIV prevention technologies [56]. Tatoud illustrates that the growing number of new HIV infections places pressure on the development of new prevention technologies, which are dependent on evidence-based policy, research, and funding. New prevention technologies, however, also depend on their uptake, which itself is mediated by access, human rights, gender equality, acceptability, and protective motivations. Addressing these ethical issues will be key to the success of TasP. The impact of TasP is also diminished by misuse, poor adherence, risk compensation, and adverse side effects. However, the effects of these diversions will not be immediately apparent. As TasP is scaled-up and if TasP reduces the number of new infections, it will relieve pressure for developing new prevention technologies. A consequence of TasP may therefore be stagnation in HIV prevention that could leave few future options should TasP not reach its expectations over the long haul.

# Chapter 2
# Reflecting on Prevention Technologies

*By condoning and embracing the concept of giving free needles to drug addicts, President Clinton has raised the white flag of surrender. Instead of leadership on the issue, we get a deadhead president who supports a program that gives free needles to drug addicts.*

*US Congressman Tom Delay (1998)*

It may not seem obvious, but behavioral interventions for HIV prevention have always hinged on medical technologies. Sterile syringes, condoms, and HIV testing are the tools of behavioral prevention. Overtime these medical devices have become fully integrated with practical skills to the point at which they are inseparable from behavior itself. We know that these tools are most effective when delivered through a broader array of services. For instance, placing a bowl of condoms in a bathhouse is less effective than social marketing strategies to promote their use. Even HIV antibody testing without risk reduction counseling is merely a medical diagnostic test with no evidence for risk reduction of its own. It is the human interphase that determines the preventive value of these technologies. As treatments become the next tool of prevention, their use will also be at the mercy of perceptions, motivations, desires, beliefs, and behaviors. Perhaps the lessons learned from biomedical HIV prevention technologies of the past can help bolster the success of TasP.

## Needles and Syringes

In the USA, injection drug use is the source of 8% of men's and 15% of women's HIV infection. HIV rapidly spreads through injection drug using networks because infected blood is highly infectious and the virus directly enters a susceptible blood stream. Even when blood plasma viral load is undetectable HIV concentrations are sufficient for transmission. Similar to sexual relationships, injection equipment is often shared within intimate and trusted relationships, inhibiting partners from taking precautions. Reducing the risk for HIV among injection drug users therefore requires both access to sterile injection equipment and changing the social dynamics of injecting drugs.

S.C. Kalichman, *HIV Treatments as Prevention (TasP):*
*Primer for Behavior-Based Implementation*, SpringerBriefs in Public Health,
DOI 10.1007/978-1-4614-5119-8_2, © Seth C. Kalichman 2013

**Fig. 2.1** Number of incident
HIV infections in New York
City injection drug users,
AJPH 1990 (Data from Des
Jarlais et al. [174] used with
permission)

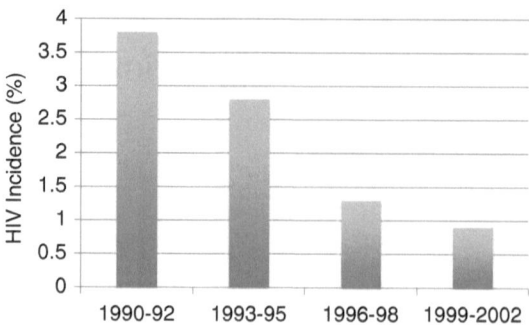

**Fig. 2.2** Number of sterile
syringes exchanged in New
York City, 1990–2002 (Data
from Des Jarlais et al. [174],
used with permission)

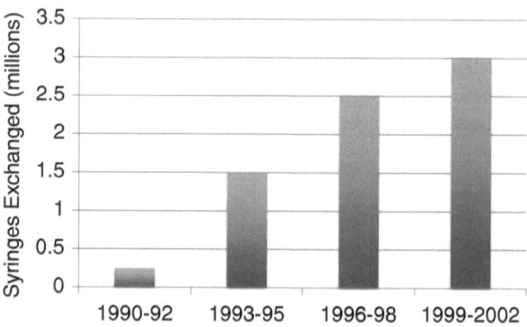

## Syringe Access

Needles and syringes are basic medical supplies and their access is a matter of
social policy. It is well known that providing injection drug users with access to
clean injection equipment prevents HIV infections. Evaluations of syringe exchange
programs demonstrate 33% reductions in HIV incidence in New Haven, 50% in
Amsterdam, and 70% in New York City [57–59]. Don Des Jarlais and his colleagues
at the Albert Einstein School of Medicine in New York City offer compelling evidence for the impact of syringe access on HIV epidemics. The number of syringes
exchanged in New York increased from under 500,000 in 1990 to over three million
in 2002. HIV incidence decreased during that same period from nearly 4% per year
to less than 1% (see Figs. 2.1 and 2.2). Hepatitis C virus (HCV) is ten times easier
to transmit through blood than is HIV, and syringe exchange programs demonstrate
significant impacts on this disease as well. In 1990 80% of HIV uninfected injection
drug users in New York were infected with HCV. Following implementation of
syringe access programs, HCV infection rates dropped off sharply to 59% in 2001.
Among persons who had been injecting for less than 6 years, the HCV infection rate
fell from 80 to 38%. These findings represent a fraction of the significant body of
research that demonstrates the public health impact of syringe access. Because the
distribution of sterile syringes is determined by public policies, legislators have
been the primary impediment to scaling up this effective strategy.

## Politics of Syringe Access

Few public health failures are as infuriating as the ban on US Federal funding for clean injection equipment. In 1988 the US Congress established a prohibition on using Federal funds to pay for clean needles and syringe access. The ban remained in place for over a decade when it seemed likely that President Clinton would correct this misguided policy. The debate over syringe access peaked in 1998 when the public health benefits of needle exchange programs became indisputable. Numerous scientists and public health experts were on the frontlines of the fight. David Vlahov, then at the New York Academy of Sciences, presented a wealth of evidence to the 1997 NIH Consensus Development Conference. He presented evaluations of needle exchange programs, many operating since 1986, that clearly saved countless lives. Vlahov relied on rigorous research conducted by Yale University's Robert Heimer and Edward Kaplan showing the incidence of HIV infections had dropped by 33% in New Haven as a direct result of private and state funded needle exchange programs. The NIH panel was briefed on research that demonstrated protective effects of needle exchange on HIV incidence in New York City. The NIH panel also heard evidence for the long-term impact of needle exchange on HIV prevalence in Chicago, Tacoma, Sydney, Toronto, and Glasgow. Every concern that justified the Federal ban was put to rest. Needle exchange does not promote drug use; in fact these programs encourage entering drug treatment. And because needles are exchanged on a one-to-one basis, they could not increase the number of needles in circulation. Research from the CDC showed that the rate of new HIV infections decreased by as much as 80% as a direct result of these programs.

Chaired by David Reiss of George Washington University Medical Center, the NIH panel determined that syringe and needle exchange programs are effective at reducing HIV infections and should be implemented with adequate resources. The panel concluded:

> Legislative restriction on needle exchange programs must be lifted because such legislation constitutes a major barrier to realizing the potential of a powerful approach and exposes millions of people to unnecessary risk..... Of utmost importance is that HIV prevention policy be based, whenever possible, on scientific information. This occurs too little—the behavior placing the public health at greatest risk may be occurring in legislative and other decision making bodies. The Federal ban on funding for needle exchange programs as well as restrictions on selling injection equipment are absolutely contraindicated and erect formidable barriers to implementing what is known to be effective. Many thousands of unnecessary deaths will occur as a result.

The NIH recommendations led to even more policy positions issued by the American Medical Association, the American Bar Association, the American Public Health Association, The Association of State and Territorial Health Officials, National Academy of Sciences, American Academy of Pediatrics, American Nurses Association, and The US Conference of Mayors. Every leading public health institute in the world declared syringe exchange a cheap and accessible biomedical device effective in preventing HIV infections.

With evidence and pressure from public health lobbies, the US Congress again debated lifting the Federal ban on funds for needle exchange programs. California representative Nancy Pelosi echoed the call for lifting the ban, stating that "Sound science is an essential component of good public policy, and the scientific support for needle exchange could not be more clear." Texas congresswoman Sheila Jackson Lee added, "Secretary of Health and Human Services, the Director of the NIH, and the National Institute on Drug Abuse issued a determination that scientific evidence indicates that needle exchange reduces HIV transmission and absolutely does not encourage the use of illegal drugs."

But public policy is not necessarily persuaded by evidence. California representative Frank Riggs summarized the support for maintaining the Federal ban on needle exchange, stating "We do not want to be in a position where we use tax payer funding or other tax revenues to promote illegal drug use, to promote further drug addiction, and drug dependency." Public health lost the debate when congress voted 287–140 to make the ban on Federal funding for needle exchange "permanent."

The ban stayed in place until July 27, 2009 when congress voted 218–211 in favor of lifting the ban. Signed by President Obama more than 15 years after research had definitively proven the effectiveness of needle exchange in preventing HIV infections. Today, US cities with the most number of syringes exchanged are the cities with the least number of new injection drug use HIV infections. The Harm Reduction Coalition lists 7-syringe access programs in New York City and 5% of HIV infections in New York in 2009 were among injection drug users. In contrast, there is only one syringe access program in Washington, DC where 28% of new infections in 2009 occurred among injection drug users.

Even the most comprehensive and expensive needle exchange programs are cost saving, documenting a return of $4 saved in health care costs for every $1 invested in needle exchange. For example, harm reduction centers and supervised facilities provide safe injection places as well as linkages to drug treatment, HIV testing, and medical care. A cost evaluation of one supervised injection facility in Vancouver British Columbia showed that HIV infections are averted at one-tenth the cost of caring for a person with HIV [10]. A more recent economic evaluation by Steve Pinkerton at the Medical College of Wisconsin showed that at an annual cost of $3 million, a supervised injection facility prevents 83 new HIV infections a year, saving $17.6 million in medical expenses [52].

The US is not the only country slow to act on needle exchange. Russia, for example, has an HIV epidemic that is fueled by contaminated injection equipment. The first documented case of AIDS in Russia occurred in St. Petersburg in the mid-1980s. Following a substantial outbreak of HIV in nearby Kaliningrad, it seemed that St. Petersburg was on the brink of an AIDS disaster [60]. At first compartmentalized among opiate injectors, heterosexual transmissions soon followed, as did a significant epidemic among Russian men who have sex with men. Oppressive drug policies, police intimidation of harm reduction and outreach workers, and homophobia hampered efforts to prevent HIV infections. Russia and the Ukraine account for 90% of all new HIV infections in Eastern Europe [22, 32]. Similar tragedies are playing out in Asia as well. The failure of policy makers to act on simple proven means for preventing HIV epidemics have brought some of the darkest days in the AIDS pandemic.

We have known since the late 1980s that syringe access is most effective when implemented within broader services. The aims of syringe access are to replace contaminated needles/syringes with clean equipment, reduce the number of contaminated syringes circulating in drug using networks, and link injection drug users to prevention and treatment services. At the 2011 meeting of the International AIDS Society, Don Des Jarlais outlined six principles of best practices for syringe exchange programs:

- Programs should be started when HIV prevalence is low to keep infections low
- Programs should be large scale with no limits on syringes and no requirement for one-to-one exchange
- Services should be provided at convenient locations and hours of operation
- Programs should provide multiple services including HIV testing, condom distribution, etc.
- Involve drug injectors as peers and experts in the site operations
- Work to ensure cooperation of law enforcement

Syringe exchange programs are further bolstered by social network interventions, again illustrating the power of integrating biomedical and behavioral prevention strategies.

## Social Interventions for Injection Drug Users

HIV is spread through sexual and drug sharing networks. Intervening at the network level offers some of the most effective interventions for reducing HIV transmission. In these programs, injectors are recruited through outreach. As part of their participation, peers recruit their friends into subsequent intervention waves. The genius of this approach is that the level of intervention is matched to the level of HIV transmission. Interventions targeting injection drug users have implicitly and explicitly infiltrated social networks through informal conversations, community-level education, and advocacy. Social network interventions have demonstrated irrefutable success in reducing injection associated HIV transmission risks and, to a lesser degree, sexual risks.

Carl Latkin at Johns Hopkins University is a pioneer in network-level interventions. Latkin and his colleagues developed the first intensive behavioral interventions aimed at injection drug using networks. These innovative programs focus on reducing injection drug use behaviors (i.e., Stop AIDS for Everybody, SAFE) and reducing sexual transmission risks (i.e., Self-Help in Eliminating Life-Threatening Diseases, SHIELD) [61–65]. In the SHIELD intervention, injection drug users meet in ten small group sessions for training in risk reduction strategies. The intervention was designed to impact the participant's own injection drug use as well as the injection practices of their network members. The intervention was designed for use in drug treatment centers, homeless shelters, and other ongoing services. Drawing from Latkin and Tobin's descriptions [66, 67], the intervention is grounded in cognitive-behavioral models of behavior change common in skills-training interventions. SHIELD provides opportunities to personalize and conceptualize the meaning of HIV-related risk behaviors. Group members are instructed in strategies for examining individual and social-level factors that influence their decisions and actions. As typically occurs in skills-based interventions, the training emphasizes interactive techniques including modeling, performance, behavioral rehearsal, feedback, and public goal setting. Role-playing and other safer sex exercises were a key strategy for increasing comfort in reducing sexual risks, especially condom use. The SHIELD intervention embraces a harm reduction orientation by providing an array of options for reducing risk behaviors.

An important feature of SHIELD is that participants make public commitments to improve their own health behaviors and promote HIV prevention within their networks. A central tenant of SHIELD is to enhance a sense of community among network members. This goal is achieved through activities that contextualize HIV within broader community concerns. SHIELD participants identified major concerns in their community and discussed how HIV impacts the people they know. Group participants were asked what they could do to reduce the spread of HIV and to address other issues in their community. Building self-determination and a sense of community, there was significant attention to the interrelatedness of individuals, risk partners, and network members. SHIELD was therefore designed to harness the power of social norms and exploit their influence on behaviors.

Group members were encouraged to carry forward HIV education within their networks and to advocate risk reduction among their sex and drug partners, family, and friends. Positive health-promoting actions were intended to replace risk behaviors, creating multiple waves of prevention within established social networks. The behavioral skills built on naturally occurring protective behaviors within existing relationships. Sam Friedman of the National Development Research Institute described these behaviors as intravention. He identified protective injection drug using networks where preventive behaviors are normative and HIV prevalence remains low [68, 69]. Freidman described individuals within protective networks engaged in altruistic actions aimed at reducing network member risks. Motivated by the relationships themselves, individuals advised their friends to avoid risk, take precautions, and support protective actions. SHIELD exploits pro-social behaviors to propagate and strengthen intravention. SHIELD participants were themselves trained in peer outreach strategies and provided with informational brochures, syringe sterilization kits, and condoms for distribution in their networks.

The outcomes from a randomized trial testing the SHIELD intervention demonstrated reductions in both injection and sexual risk behaviors. Participants in SHIELD decreased injecting drugs 6 months after the intervention; 48% of SHIELD group members had decreased injecting compared to 25% of the control participants. It was common for participants to completely cease injecting drugs, with 44% of SHIELD participants and 22% of control participants stopping their drug use. In all, 69% of SHIELD group members no longer used unhygienic needles compared to 30% of control participants. In a multivariate analysis that controlled for multiple confounding factors including age, gender, race, education, arrest history, HIV status, and mood, the SHIELD group was more than three times likely to report stopping injection drug use and reducing needle sharing.

With respect to sexual risk reduction, 16% of SHIELD group members increased their condom use during vaginal sex with casual partners compared to only 4% of those in the control group. The SHIELD participants were more than seven times as likely to report increased use of condoms with casual partners. In addition, 18% of persons in the SHIELD groups reduced their number of casual sex partners compared to 7% of controls. These findings dovetail with reductions in injection risks to demonstrate multiple preventive benefits of the SHIELD intervention.

SHIELD builds on the success of earlier network-level interventions for injection drug users that focused solely on needle sharing and other drug-related risks. The intervention was innovative in its integration of both drug use and sexual risk behavior change in a single model. In that sense, SHIELD foreshadows the integration of multiple combinations of interventions that forms the state of HIV prevention today.

## Condoms

The first cases of AIDS rather quickly revealed that the cause was sexually transmitted. Condoms became the first line of defense against AIDS even before HIV was discovered. The biomedical principle behind barrier methods is simple; placing an impermeable membrane between the virus and vulnerable cells will prevent infection. Two barrier methods have proven successful for HIV prevention—male condoms and female condoms.

While condoms prevent HIV infections, getting people to use them has proven to be the great challenge in HIV prevention. A fundamental truth in HIV prevention is that people hold two desires—to feel safe and to not use condoms. When used correctly and consistently, condoms provide nearly perfect protection against HIV. Condoms rarely fail in preventing STI, but we have failed to exploit their preventive benefits. Thousands of studies throughout the world show that attitudes toward condoms offset the protection they offer. The new standard in HIV prevention is to all but dismiss condoms. Condoms have been replaced with partner selection strategies, negotiating safety, and avoiding certain sexual positions; choices that help people feel safer with little safety.

### *Male Condoms*

Condoms are the least expensive and most widely available means of preventing HIV. An industry report estimates that by 2016 the global market will reach 27 billion condoms. In South Africa, the country with the world's largest AIDS epidemic, condoms are ubiquitous. The South African Department of Health distributes more than 400 million condoms annually and millions of additional condoms are doled out by non-governmental organizations. The Treatment Action Campaign, for example, provides more than one million condoms each month in the Western Cape Province alone.

Unless they break, slip-off, or are not used at all, condoms offer nearly complete protection against the spread of HIV. Laboratory testing shows that latex condoms are not easily broken. Condoms can be pumped with air to the size of a watermelon without bursting. Air and water burst tests show that more than 99% of condoms do not leak. Even when condoms do leak, they reduce exposure to HIV by a factor of more than 10,000 times. In practice, condom breakage rates fall between 1 and 10%, with user errors caused by insufficient lubrication, improper lubrication with oil-based products, reuse, excessive strain, and slippage.

Condom failure can also occur from incorrect use, such as leaving an insufficient reservoir at the tip or leaving excessive air bubbles in the condom. In the USA, contraceptive condom failures are as high as 17% annually [70]. In one study of adolescents, Rick Crosby and his colleagues found that as many as one in three sexually active youth experience condom failures, which are associated with subsequent STI [71]. In a study of STI clinic patients in Cape Town, South Africa we found 37% of men and 41% of women report lifetime histories of condom failures. We also found that oil-based lubricants were a factor in 12% of persons experiencing condom failure [72]. But the real problem is not the condoms themselves, but rather getting people to use them.

Consistent condom use means using one every time a person has sex, from start to finish. In reality, intermittent condom use is far more common. Condom use generally increases after a rise in HIV prevalence. For example, condom use reported during last intercourse among men who have sex with men in China was 56% in 2003–2005, increasing to 61% between 2006 and 2008, paralleling increased HIV prevalence in the population [73]. Increases in condom use are understandably reactive to rising HIV prevalence, which of course is too late for primary prevention.

Attitudes, beliefs, and perceptions ultimately determine condom use. Most negative attitudes toward condoms center on their interference with sexual sensation, pleasure, and sexual intimacy. Condoms can also become associated with disease and distrust. Less studied are the physiological aspects of sexual response in relation to condoms. Jeff Kelly and I suggested in 1995 that condom use should be placed in the realm of emotion and sexual arousal rather than reasoning and rational decision-making [74].

Early efforts in HIV prevention focused on increasing condom use by directly addressing negative attitudes. In fact, the very first behavioral HIV prevention interventions were primarily aimed at eroticizing condoms. Ribbed surfaces, exotic scents, and vibrant colors were combined with a cornucopia of lubricants to accentuate sensuality. These products certainly brought variety and choice. Although met with initial enthusiasm, there is little evidence that these products have done much to sustain condom use.

To directly address the sensation problem, manufacturers started making condoms from materials other than latex. Most promising were condoms made of polyurethane, a thin, durable plastic. It seemed that a plastic condom could be marketed in direct response to the growing resistance against latex. My research team conducted a study aimed at testing the uptake of polyurethane male condoms. We designed a 3-h workshop to encourage men to use polyurethane condoms. Men were told, "everyone knows rubbers can ruin the moment, but new plastic condoms are different." Polyurethane condoms are thinner and men were told that the plastic allowed heat to transfer in both directions. The fact that polyurethane condoms do not grip the penis was also talked-up as an advantage. Despite our best efforts, the intervention did not lead to men beating down the door for polyurethane condoms. Men did use the polyurethane condoms, but they used latex condoms less. The net result was little change in protection.

Many other efforts to increase condom use have failed. For example, there are devices that assist men in rolling condoms on. There is also a spray-on condom, where the penis is inserted in to a hard plastic tube with interior nozzles that spray liquid latex in all directions, like water jets in a car wash. Another innovation to get people to use condoms is a product called Futura—a condom laced with a vasodilating gel to boost penile blood flow and maintain erections. Dubbed a Viagra condom, the idea is to increase appeal of using condoms by making sex with condoms last longer. None of these products have shown evidence of overcoming the power of negative attitudes.

## Politics of Condoms

In May of 1988 the US Surgeon General C. Everett Koop released his report on AIDS to America. The report remains the largest dissemination of public health information in US history, with 107 million copies mailed to US households. The Surgeon General provided facts, telling us what we could do to avoid AIDS and just as importantly, what we did not need to be concerned about. Upon reflection, Koop reveals, "Of all the things I said, only two words seemed to be remembered: sex education, and the next few days were spent fending off press questions about when sex education should begin, and all the questions that come to mind if your interest is in sex education. Many of the issues of AIDS in the report seemed eclipsed by this distraction" [75].

The problem is how we define "sex education." Comprehensive approaches embrace sexuality in a developmental context and address all aspects of sexual health and behaviors. In contrast, narrow approaches to sex education typically focus on abstinence. Advocacy for abstinence only sex education is firmly grounded in religious and political ideologies. In the parallel universe that saw syringe access voted down in the US Congress, the debate regarding comprehensive versus abstinence only sex education is not settled by evidence.

In 1996, President Clinton signed the Public Health Service Act, Public Law 104-193 to award States block grants for programs targeting HIV prevention for adolescents. However, the designated funds could only be used for abstinence education. Even at that time there was evidence that abstinence programs don't work. The NIH Consensus Conference showed that comprehensive sex education is our best means of protecting the sexual health of young people. The NIH Panel noted that the new Federal policies were not in synch with the science and concluded:

> The single greatest increase in HIV prevention funding occurred with 1996 Federal legislation in the United States providing $50 million within block grant entitlements for programs teaching adolescents abstinence from sexual behavior. Among the criteria for programs funded through the block grant program are the following two requirements: (a) 'has as its exclusive purpose, teaching the social psychological, and health gains to be realized by abstaining from sexual activity' and (b) 'teaches that a mutually faithful monogamous relationship in the context of marriage is the expected standard of human sexual activity' (Public Health Service Act, Public Law 104-193, Sec. 912). Some programs based on an abstinence model propose that approaches such as the use of condoms are ineffective. This model places policy in direct conflict with science because it ignores overwhelming evidence that other programs are effective. Abstinence-only programs cannot be justified in the face of effective programs and given the fact that we face an international emergency in the AIDS epidemic (available at http://consensus.nih.gov/1997/1997PreventHIVRisk104PDF.pdf).

Today the research could not be any clearer. There is no evidence that abstinence only sex education programs achieve their goals. For example one study randomly assigned adolescents to one of four-abstinence programs or a control group [76]. The programs defined as abstinence-only had the following key characteristics:

- Have as its exclusive purpose teaching the social, psychological, and health gains to be realized by abstaining from sexual activity.
- Teach abstinence from sexual activity outside marriage as the expected standard for all school-age children.
- Teach that abstinence from sexual activity is the only certain way to avoid out-of-wedlock pregnancy, sexually transmitted diseases, and other associated health problems.
- Teach that a mutually faithful, monogamous relationship in the context of marriage is the expected standard of sexual activity.
- Teach that sexual activity outside the context of marriage is likely to have harmful psychological and physical effects.
- Teach that bearing children out of wedlock is likely to have harmful consequences for the child, the child's parents, and society.
- Teach young people how to reject sexual advances and how alcohol and drug use increase vulnerability to sexual advances.
- Teach the importance of attaining self-sufficiency before engaging in sexual activity.

While teens that received the abstinence programs did acquire accurate information about STI and contraception, the improved knowledge did not lead to behavior change. There were no differences in sexual behaviors observed in this study. In the end, 56% of adolescents who received abstinence education remained abstinent after the program, as did 55% of those in the control group. As much as 78 months later, 49% were abstinent regardless of which program they received [77]. In another randomized controlled trial, John Jemmott and his colleagues tested three-structured and manual-based brief interventions for adolescents: (a) an evidence-based safer sex program called "Be Proud—Be Responsible," (b) an abstinence only program, or (c) a time-matched non-sexual health program to serve as the control group. Importantly, the abstinence intervention had a similar tone as the safer sex program, to avoid portraying sex in a negative light or send any moralistic messages. The results were clear. One year after the program, 20% of the abstinence program participants had engaged in sex, as did 16.5% of the safer sex participants and 23% of the control group. Direct comparisons showed that the safer sex intervention resulted in significantly less unprotected sex than the other two programs.

Scientific evidence and public health aside, President George W. Bush further promoted abstinence only sex education. The official US policy was to promote an approach to HIV prevention known as the ABCs—Abstinence, Be Faithful, and Condoms. However, the seeds of abstinence only prevention were shown more than a decade earlier during the Regan Administration. President Reagan's Surgeon General Koop stated "I never mentioned the use of condoms as a preventive measure against AIDS without first stressing the much better—and much safer—alternatives of abstinence and/or monogamy" [75].

The ABC mantra became a congressional mandate for funding HIV prevention, both domestically and internationally [78]. Because all US HIV prevention activities were required to embrace the ABC approach, the CDC went so far as to require all of its evidence-based prevention packages to include a back-tab in the manual for a standard ABC curriculum guide. Ironically, none of the "evidence" based interventions were even remotely related to an ABC approach and there are no such interventions that have been demonstrated effective [79]. Once again, AIDS prevention science fell on deaf ears.

## *Condom Counseling*

Behavioral interventions can concentrate on multiple avenues to HIV prevention including reducing numbers of partners, abstaining from high-risk practices, or reducing substance use in sexual contexts. But every behavioral risk reduction intervention of value has included increasing condom use. Increased condom use is typically greater in casual than committed relationships. Condoms are also used more with known HIV-infected partners than non-infected partners. Meta-analyses show that increased condom use is among the most consistent behavioral intervention outcomes. Interventions delivered in individual counseling, small groups, or at the community level have all demonstrated increases in condom use. While interventions vary widely, they share much in common when it comes to promoting condom use. Changing negative attitudes toward condoms is an explicit aim of risk reduction counseling. However, purely cognitive approaches to increasing condom use are criticized for ignoring the physiological, sensation, and emotional aspects of sexual experience. Eroticizing condoms usually takes a hands-on approach by touching and feeling lubricated latex, placing condoms on anatomic models, and planning to incorporate condom use in the heat of the moment.

One key feature of interactive activities is condom desensitization. An HIV prevention intervention is perhaps the only time that a person will handle a condom in the light. It may also be the only time they will discuss the pros and cons of condoms. The experience also offers the opportunity to self-reflect and to consider the trade-off between increased protections versus loss of sensation. Although we do not know exactly what behavior change mechanisms are at work in condom skills training, it is likely they go beyond the technical accuracies of proper condom use.

## Condom Successes

Condoms are effective at preventing the spread of disease at the individual and population levels. Aside from clean needles and syringes, no other prevention technology has thus far demonstrated a direct correspondence between access, uptake, and disease prevention. For example, Fig. 2.3 shows the relationship between condom distribution and STI rates in one South African township. The data illustrate peaks in condom distribution that coincide with declining rates of STI. The rises and falls in condom distribution suggest variations in supply or demand. Condoms distributed by the City of Cape Town Health Department are more a function of restocking clinics than implementing any particular program.

Coordinated efforts to distribute and promote condoms have proven successful in reducing disease. The best-known example is Thailand's 100% Condom Program discussed earlier. This program embedded a broad-based approach to achieving 100% condom use among Thai military conscripts [80, 81]. The program included chaplains and medics delivering STI and condom use education, including a series of mandatory weekly discussions. Information on STI prevention was distributed along with scaled-up access to condoms. Small group workshops were also implemented to deliver intensive communication skills, condom use skills, role-plays, social reinforcement, and other behavioral strategies. Condoms were distributed using social marketing techniques. The results were impressive, with military recruits assigned to the program demonstrating 75% fewer HIV infections and 85% reductions in other STI compared to men who did not receive the program.

Thailand instituted a broader social policy for condom distribution that targeted high-risk populations. These efforts are widely recognized for reversing what was clearly an emerging AIDS crisis in Thailand. Mike Merson, former Director of the World Health Organization's Global AIDS Program, described the program as:

> The best evaluated effort of a nationwide program in a developing country has been that of Thailand, and it demonstrates the value of combining intervention approaches. In that country, where the commercial sex industry is well established, a mass condom promotional campaign was begun in the late 1980s and a 100-percent condom use program was

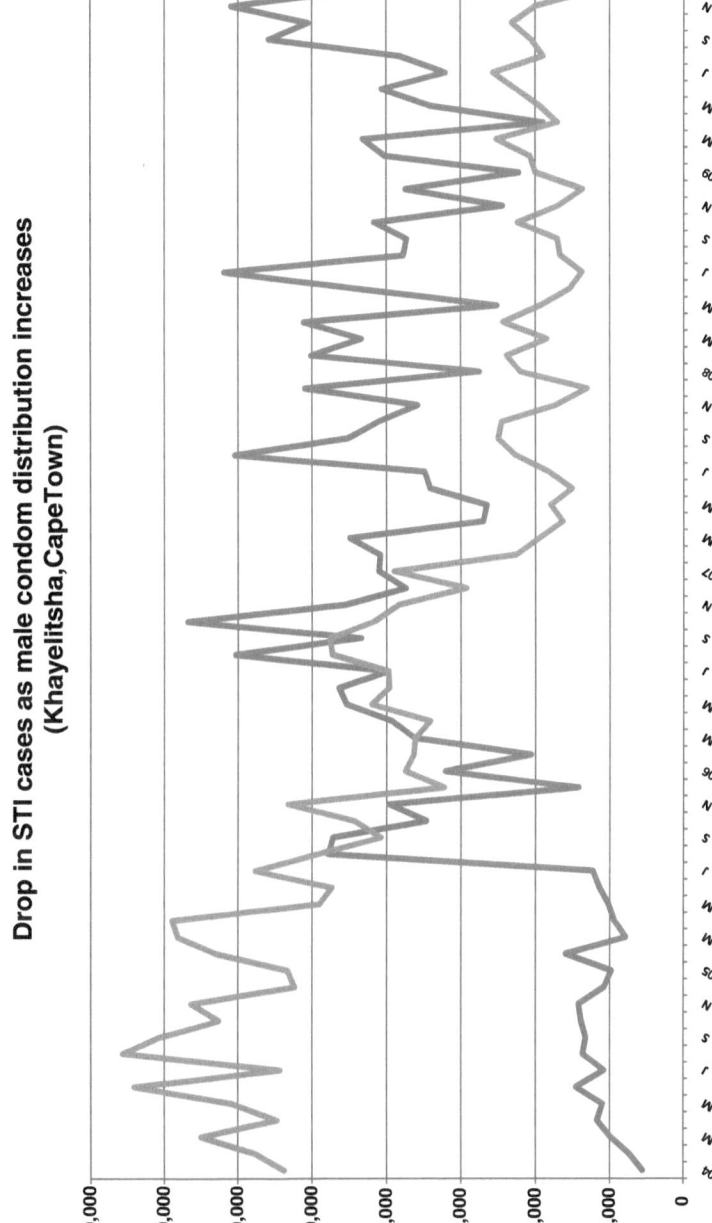

**Fig. 2.3** Relationship between condom distribution and STI rates in a Cape Town South African township (*Source*: The City of Cape Town Department of Health)

instituted in brothels in northern Thailand in 1989 and in the entire country early in 1992. Antibiotics are also readily available for treatment of STDs. These together resulted in a more than six-fold increase in the percentage of sex acts with commercial sex workers in which a condom was used, from 14 percent before 1989 to over 90 percent in December 1994, with a concomitant decrease of 85 percent in male STD cases nationwide seen at government clinics and a decline in HIV prevalence in pregnant women and military conscripts by the end of this period. This impact has been most vividly demonstrated in northern Thailand, where there has been a significant decrease in HIV prevalence among military conscripts from 12.5 percent in 1991 to 6.7 percent in 1995 [82].

HIV incidence in Thailand peaked in 1995 and has since declined. The country's aggressive prevention policies extended beyond scaling-up condom promotion to include syringe access, testing, and treatment. But there is no question that the 100% condom program had an impact.

## *Condom Double Standards*

The standard for success of condoms is that one be used every time a person has sex—complete and consistent use. Using condoms during less than every sex act is generally considered a failure. But only condoms are held to a standard of perfect protection. Other prevention technologies, including vaccines, microbicides, and TasP are deemed successful with 40% protection. Male circumcision is considered a success because it can permanently cut HIV transmission in half. We are elated when a vaginal microbicide reduces HIV infections by 35% and thrilled when PrEP reduced HIV infections by 45%. No one expects any HIV prevention technology other than condoms to completely protect against HIV. For example, the FDA has suggested that condom packages include the following statement, "when used correctly and every time you have sex, latex condoms greatly reduce, but do not eliminate the risk of catching or spreading HIV, the virus that causes AIDS."

Interventions that demand 100% condom use are set up to fail. On the other hand, interventions that aspire to increase condom use beyond some critical level, say 50% protection, are realistic. Several behavioral interventions have demonstrated meaningful increases in condom use. In one trial, Gina Wingood and her colleagues at Emory University reported that more than twice as many women who received a group prevention intervention reported consistent condom use than women in a control condition 1 year later [83]. However considerable protection was afforded to women who did not use condoms every time they had sex; a mean of 76% of intercourse occasions were condom protected among women in the intervention group compared to a mean of 54% for the comparison group. Tom Patterson at the University of California at San Diego reported similar findings from an intervention for female sex workers in Mexico, with average condom use increasing from 56 to 83% of intercourse occasions protected and increased condom use coincided with a 40% decline in STI. Even when inconsistent or incomplete, condom use translates to greater protection, usually exceeding the typically aspired level of 35% risk reduction.

## Where Have All the Condoms Gone?

Condoms are the frontline defense against HIV infection. In 1995 there were over 450 million condoms sold in the USA. In 2010, the global condom market was worth nearly $4 billion and is expected to exceed $6 billion by 2015. And yet the demand outpaces the supply. With 16 million sexually active men in South Africa, the 450 million condoms distributed each year amounts to about 28 condoms per man. Condom shortages are becoming frighteningly common in many developing countries, especially those with the greatest HIV prevalence. Non-governmental organizations in China started providing free condoms to men who have sex with men after homosexuality was decriminalized in 1997. Nevertheless, over 16% of men who have sex with men in China state that condoms are unavailable [73].

According to the United Nations Population Fund, condom supplies have not met demand in developing countries since 1996. In 2005, at least 13.1 billion condoms were needed to reduce the spread of HIV in developing countries and yet only 2.3 billion were donated in 2005 and 3.4 billion in 2007. On average, African countries receive about ten condoms per man each year, whereas developing countries outside of Africa receive as few as one condom per man. Throughout Africa, studies of venues where people meet sex partners show that fewer than half have condoms available [84].

Shortages of female condoms are also common. International shipments of female condoms grew from 1.1 million in 2003 to over 14 million in 2009. The USA is a major donor of female condoms to developing countries providing 40% of female condoms sent to developing countries. Yet, female condoms only account for 3% of US condom shipments. Although the demand for female condoms varies, news reports suggest shortages in high-HIV prevalence countries [85]. It is challenging enough to get people to use condoms and short supplies are not helping. Given the cost differentials, condom shortages paint a bleak picture for TasP with much more dire consequences.

## Female Condoms

Gender-power differentials in sexual relationships place women at-risk for HIV and were at the core of developing the female condom. Often described as a vaginal liner, there are a variety of such products available. Some female condoms have an internal framework of sponges that help anchor the lining in place. Other variations use panties to hold a replaceable liner in place. Perhaps the most elaborate model consists of a polyurethane pouch that is packaged inside a film capsule inserted in the vagina. The capsule dissolves, leaving four small foam forms that serve as anchors on the outside of a pouch. The idea behind all female condoms is to shift the initiation and a great degree of control for condom use from men to women. Female condoms require a minimal amount of cooperation from male sex partners [86].

The Female Health Company produces the most familiar female condom. Indeed, this product has been branded "The Female Condom" and it has almost universally been the subject of research. First approved by the FDA in 1993 as a contraceptive, the female condom soon demonstrated efficacy for preventing STI, including HIV. Female condom effectiveness research mirrors that of male condoms. Studies testing the vagina for post-coital markers show traces of semen in 17% of female condom users compared to 14% for male condoms. Female condoms break and tear at lower rates than male condoms, failing approximately 1% of the time. Female condom use reduces the probability of HIV transmission by as much as 97% [87]. To help manage the cost of female condoms, there are instructions for cleaning and reuse up to five times. However, the female condom is not without complaints including cost, which is typically between 35¢ and 55¢, compared to the 3¢ for male condoms. Women also complain about insertion difficulties and crinkling noises during sex. To address these concerns, there is a second generation of less expensive and quieter synthetic latex female condoms. Released in 2009, the new female condom revitalized efforts to promote its use.

With high expectations that it would revolutionize contraception and STI prevention, female condoms have generated considerable interest and discussion. The female condom is mostly acceptable to both women and men. However, women often use female condoms with just one sex partner. There is also evidence that the female condom is used mostly out of curiosity. Women who are already infected with HIV demonstrate greater use than women at-risk for HIV infection. Negative attitudes toward female condoms are more common among women who have not yet used them [87]. For example, 82% of women living with HIV who have never used a female condom do not believe they feel better than male condoms and 54% say the female condom is difficult to use. Negative attitudes may be hard to change if they keep women from even trying female condoms.

Although the female condom is intended to shift power dynamics in sexual decisions, it does not appear that they have succeeded. A challenge to female condom use is once again resistance from male partners. Male partners' reactions to the female condom predict their use [87]. Many women do not choose to use female condoms because they fear negative reactions and objections of their male partners. Women may also not want to diminish the sex roles of men. Women who initiate female condom use can experience the same risks for adverse reactions and violence that they have experienced when suggesting their partners use male condoms [88].

For women who do try female condoms, they may replace male condoms. Product substitution in this case would have no impact on protection given the nearly equal preventive value of male and female condoms. However, there is evidence that the female condom is used in situations where male condom use would not occur, and therefore yielding a net protective benefit [87]. Also, women are not the only ones using female condoms, with some men using the "female condom" with same sex anal intercourse partners [89].

With high-acceptability and appeal for the female condom, it is surprising they are not in greater demand. An FDA study in 2002, nearly a decade after the female condom was approved, showed less than 2% of women in the USA had ever used a female condom. In 2008, a British study found that only 1% of women had used a female condom. In a study of HIV positive women, my research team found that despite generally positive attitudes toward female condoms, only 16% of women had used one, and only 6% used them as much as they used male condoms [90]. Aggressive social marketing campaigns can increase female condom use. In Zimbabwe, for example, female condom use increased from 400,000 to more than two million in 2008. Zimbabwe had been the site of a multifaceted program aimed to increase female condom use across all sectors of women [91]. For context, UNAIDS reported in 2009 more than 50 million women used female condoms worldwide.

The low uptake of female condoms is likely the result of multiple factors, including a lack of interest in long-term use. Such was our experience in South African STI clinics, where nurses complained that they could not access the female condom because of their cost. We started bringing the clinic suitcases of female condoms, usually a thousand at a time. A few years later we noticed that the clinic had a stockpile of female condoms. Supplies ramped up and demand dropped off. Ultimately, the nurses asked us to stop bringing them. It turns out that women expressed interest in the female condom, took some with them and did not return for more. The female condom intrigued women, but their use was not sustained. It would seem that female condom uptake is driven by a novelty effect.

Interventions designed to promote female condoms typically train women in their use. However, these interventions have also had disappointing results. My research team tested the effects of a 3-h workshop designed to educate women about female condoms, motivate women to use them, and build behavioral skills for bringing female condoms into sexual relationships [92]. The results showed few women used female condoms after initially trying them. It was rare for women to request more free female condoms after the intervention. In a more recent study, Theresa Hoke and her colleagues tested an intervention for female sex workers in Madagascar [93]. A total of 901 women were randomized to either receive peer education only or peer education supplemented with individual clinic-based counseling to increase male and female condom use. Results showed that there were no significant differences between conditions in male or female condom use and there were no differences between groups in aggregated STI prevalence.

## HIV Antibody Testing

HIV testing is a medical diagnostic test, not too different from cholesterol screening and mammography. In preventive medicine, diagnostic screening is aimed toward detecting disease and, when disease is detected, providing medical interventions. Just like other diagnostics, the goal of HIV testing is therefore to detect infection. Early detection increases access to medical care during critical periods of disease progression. There is also evidence that testing HIV positive has a preventive benefit. As many as half of HIV-infected people in the USA are believed to be

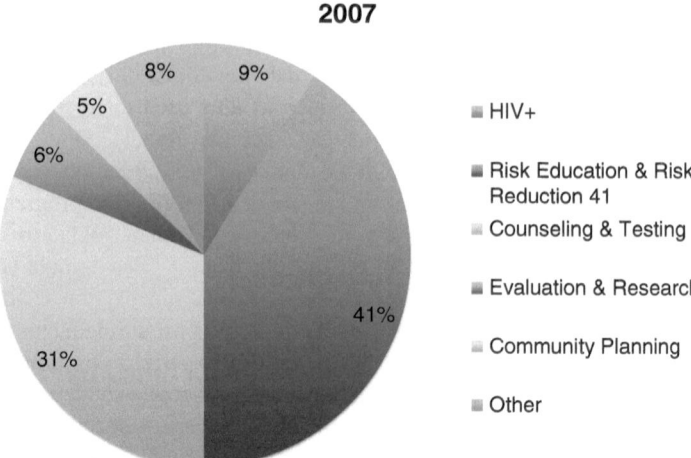

**Fig. 2.4**  CDC annual HIV prevention budget for 2007

unaware of their HIV status and are therefore unknowingly spreading the virus. The HIV transmission rate for individuals who know they are HIV positive is between 1.7 and 2.4%, whereas the rate for HIV positive persons unaware of their infection is 8.8–10.8%. HIV-infected persons who do not know their HIV status account for between 54 and 70% of new HIV infections; conversely persons who know they are infected accounted for 30–46% of infections [94]. A significant minority of HIV-infected people who transmit HIV to drug using and sex partners is the focus of TasP. In contrast, there is no apparent preventive value of HIV testing for uninfected persons, unless the testing is accompanied by a risk reduction intervention.

## Diagnostic Testing Is Not a Prevention Strategy

HIV testing itself is not a prevention strategy for uninfected persons. Testing HIV negative does not signal the need for risk reduction any more than low cholesterol tests lead to dietary changes or negative mammograms increase breast self-examination. Nevertheless, policy makers have been led to believe that HIV testing is a prevention strategy. More than half of the CDC's HIV prevention budget is dedicated to HIV testing, and that proportion is growing. Figure 2.4 shows the proportional allocation of CDC's annual HIV prevention budget in 2007, illustrating the significant increase in resources dedicated to HIV testing. As shown in Fig. 2.5 the CDC increased its funding for HIV testing in 2010 from 31% of its annual budget to 53%, which included an expansion of $143 million for new testing initiatives. At the same time, CDC removed provisions for requiring risk reduction counseling with testing, essentially gutting its potential preventive benefits.

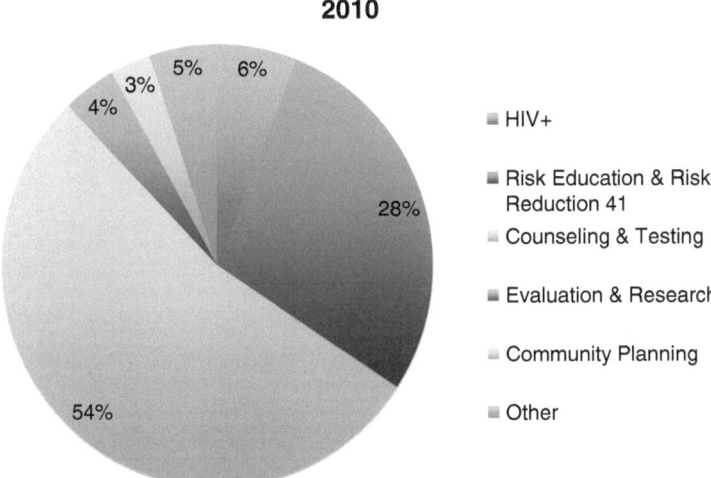

**Fig. 2.5** CDC annual HIV prevention budget for 2010

In the early years of the HIV epidemic, testing was coupled with risk reduction counseling. Beginning in 1985, the newly developed HIV antibody test was used to screen and protect blood supplies, which all but eliminated transfusion-related HIV infections. By 1987 HIV testing was recognized as an opportunity for risk reduction counseling. The CDC established standards of care for conducting client-centered counseling in conjunction with HIV testing. Client-centered counseling in the context of testing is efficient, requiring less than 30-min of pretest and posttest counseling. Historically, risk reduction counseling was an integral part of testing, but not anymore.

## Remembering Project Respect

In 1998 the CDC conducted a study to definitively answer the question, "does HIV testing and counseling reduce risks for HIV infection?" At that time behavioral interventions were still held to a standard where impact on STI would be considered compelling evidence for efficacy. Project Respect is among the most rigorously controlled HIV prevention intervention trials ever conducted. There were three main conditions to which STI clinic patients were randomized. Heterosexual men and women were tested for HIV and either received (a) two 20-min sessions of risk reduction counseling, one before and one after HIV testing that assessed personal risks for HIV, identified barriers to behavior change, developed an achievable risk reduction plan, and support patients to reduce their risks, (b) four sessions of enhanced counseling that concentrated on skills for consistent condom use and

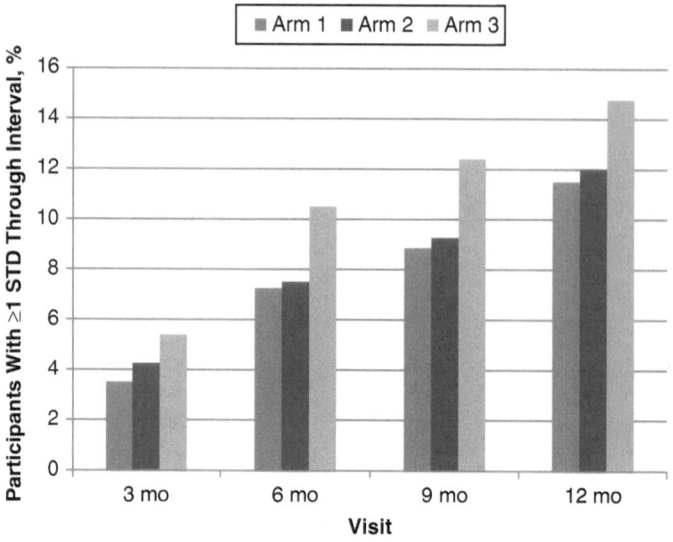

**Fig. 2.6** Incident STI over 1-year follow-up in Project Respect. Arm 1 = Standard HIV testing and counseling, Arm 2 = enhanced HIV testing and counseling, Arm 3 = HIV testing and didactic messages control (Kamb et al. [21] used with permission)

refusing to have sex without condoms; or (c) didactic prevention messages such as "be sure to use a condom," representing a minimal approach to HIV prevention. The didactic message condition included a subsample that was not assessed as often as other study conditions to examine whether the assessments themselves had an impact on behavior.

The results of Project Respect were clear. Examining the clinical records of the participating STI clinics over a year after counseling showed that 12% of patients who received the two-session counseling and 11.5% of those in the four-session counseling condition had contracted a new STI. These rates were not different from each other, but both were significantly lower than the 14.6% new infections observed in the didactic message condition (see Fig. 2.6). The greatest degree of reductions in STI were observed in the sixth month after counseling, where there were 30% fewer STI in the counseling condition than the didactic messages condition [21].

Project Respect established a new standard for HIV prevention. Many have considered the two-session counseling and testing intervention as the standard of care. David Holtgrave at Johns Hopkins University has pointed out that the CDC's press release announcing the Project Respect outcomes set the stage for its brand of client-centered counseling to become the standard of care, stating:

- "This study showed that it's not *how much* you talk to people about HIV prevention that matters most—but how you talk to them…"
- "According to CDC, the brief sessions used in this study…are feasible to implement in busy health care settings"

- "In this study, the approach was implemented with existing clinic staff, in not much more time than that required for didactic messages, and cost only eight additional dollars per client to implement"
- "Far too often, prevention programs found to be ideal in research are too difficult and expensive to implement in the real world, with this program, the ideal can be real, with few additional resources"

It seemed then that the CDC was convinced that HIV testing and counseling would prevent infections. Since 1998, new interventions are typically tested against the Project Respect testing and counseling protocol. And yet today, Project Respect is not the standard of care in practice. It is bizarre that the CDC, after great expense and effort to conduct the trial in the first place, removed requirements that HIV testing include risk reduction counseling. The CDC has reduced what may be the most effective HIV prevention intervention they had to a diagnostic test. This decision tells us much about how the highest levels of CDC policy makers view behavioral interventions. If you consider Project Respect a vision of the future, a true integration of a behavioral intervention (risk reduction counseling) with a biomedical technology (HIV testing), the implications of dismantling HIV counseling and testing does not bode well for the future of TasP.

## *The Death of Client-Centered Counseling*

Table 2.1 shows the evolution of HIV testing and counseling in past generations of the CDC's HIV testing guidelines [95]. In 2006 the CDC revised again its guidelines for HIV testing in health care settings, essentially delinking risk reduction counseling from testing. The new CDC guidelines have "acknowledged that prevention counseling is desirable for all persons at-risk for HIV but recognized that such counseling might not be appropriate or feasible in all settings." The guidelines explicitly state that the new approach does not modify standards for nonclinical settings where risk reduction counseling is less likely, such as street outreach, bath houses, festivals, and malls. Rather than maintaining a policy to improve the feasibility of risk reduction counseling, the CDC abandoned prevention counseling in health care settings, removing the hope for a preventive benefit of HIV testing beyond detecting persons already infected. The new policy specifically states:

- HIV screening is recommended for patients in all health care settings after the patient is notified that testing will be performed unless the patient declines (opt-out screening).
- Persons at high risk for HIV infection should be screened for HIV at least annually.
- Separate written consent for HIV testing should not be required; general consent for medical care should be considered sufficient to encompass consent for HIV testing.
- Prevention counseling should not be required with HIV diagnostic testing or as part of HIV screening programs in health care settings.

**Table 2.1** Evolution of CDC's HIV antibody testing guidelines 1987–2001(adapted from Phillips et al. [95])

| | 1987 | 1994 | 2001 |
|---|---|---|---|
| *Goals and scopes* | | | |
| Primary goals of testing | (1) Behavior change a primary focus (2) Identify HIV status | (1) Behavior change a primary focus (2) Identify HIV status | (1) Continued emphasis on behavior change. (2) More emphasis on identifying HIV status. |
| Scope of recommendations | Publicly funded sites | Publicly funded sites | All providers. |
| *Whether testing should be routine or targeted* | | | |
| Routinely offered to all members of a population or targeted to specific members based on risk screening | Primarily targeted | Primarily targeted | More emphasis on routine testing in high-risk and high-prevalence settings. Continued targeted testing in low prevalence settings. |
| *Informed consent* | | | |
| Whether testing is routine with informed right of referral ("opt-out" w/verbal consent only); or patients must explicitly accept or refuse testing ("opt-in" w/written consent required or recommended) | Opt-in | Opt-in | Opt-in. |
| *Information and counseling* | | | |
| Whether prevention counseling is routinely recommended | Yes | Yes | Yes for high risk settings, but risk screening recommended in other settings to determine whether counseling is recommended. |
| Relative emphasis on provision of information about HIV test, HIV transmission, and meaning of results | Information an important emphasis of pretest counseling | Information important but not a substitute for prevention counseling | Information important but not a substitute for prevention counseling. |
| Whether disclosure of results and counseling for HIV negatives should be in-person | In-person implied | In-person | Phone counseling an option. |

The CDC's rationale behind the policy change was based on two flawed lines of reasoning. First, the 2006 Guidelines state "Prevention strategies that incorporate universal HIV screening have been highly effective." However, the two cases offered to make this point are universal screening of the blood supply which has "nearly eliminated transfusion-associated HIV infection in the United States" and routine testing of pregnant women for preventing perinatal HIV transmission. Both examples speak to the value of testing as a diagnostic screening linked to broader prevention strategies—removing contaminated blood from the supply chain and administering antiretroviral medications to prevent mother-to-child transmission. In their guidelines, the CDC does not offer any evidence that universal HIV testing itself is an effective prevention strategy.

The second line of reasoning for abandoning prevention counseling with testing stems from what the CDC views as the questionable efficacy of risk reduction counseling. Specifically, the CDC states in their rationale for the new guidelines:

> The benefit of providing prevention counseling in conjunction with HIV testing is less clear. HIV counseling with testing has been demonstrated to be an effective intervention for HIV-infected participants, who increased their safer behaviors and decreased their risk behaviors; HIV counseling and testing as implemented in the studies had little effect on HIV-negative participants. However, randomized controlled trials have demonstrated that the nature and duration of prevention counseling might influence its effectiveness. Carefully controlled, theory-based prevention counseling in STD clinics has helped HIV-negative participants reduce their risk behaviors compared with participants who received only a didactic prevention message from health-care providers. A more intensive intervention among HIV-negative MSM at high risk, consisting of ten theory-based individual counseling sessions followed by maintenance sessions every 3 months, resulted in reductions in unprotected sex with partners who were HIV infected or of unknown status, compared with MSM who received structured prevention counseling only twice yearly.

Thus, the CDC's logic goes something like this: risk reduction counseling can be effective but has not been implemented according to standards and is therefore not effective. Concluding that counseling and testing failed to reduce risk was primarily based on a dated meta-analysis of HIV testing and counseling studies. Lance Weinhardt and his colleagues reviewed studies that had evaluated the impact of HIV testing and counseling on subsequent risk behavior. They found that people who test HIV positive do reduce their risk behaviors after receiving test results, but the reduction is not universal and is often not sustained. More to the point, people who test HIV negative show no evidence of reducing their risk. However, Weinhardt et al. never suggested that counseling and testing is ineffective for HIV prevention. To the contrary, they pointed to inadequate implementation and operations, all of which occurred prior to Project Respect, as the likely explanation of the poor outcomes. They concluded:

> HIV-CT (counseling and testing), at least as it was implemented in the studies reviewed, does not appear to be an effective intervention for the primary prevention of HIV infection. HIV-negative individuals did not reduce their risk behavior relative to untested participants, after HIV-CT. However, because inadequate attention has been paid to the psychological and social contexts of testing, the theoretical grounding of counseling, and the type and amount of counseling provided, a closer examination of these factors may reveal that HIV-CT is effective with HIV negative individuals under some circumstances.

It is well established by the CDC itself through Project Respect that risk reduction can be effective when it adheres to the principles of client-centered counseling. But the CDC never seriously implemented client-centered counseling as a standard of care in public or private health services. Resources have never been adequately allocated for training, quality assurance, or monitoring of risk reduction counseling. The didactic message condition in Project Respect is more consistent with counseling people currently receive with HIV testing. In fact, today the CDC has de-emphasized counseling to the point where most testing does not include hardly any prevention measures for those who test HIV negative.

In the 2006 HIV Testing Guidelines, the CDC is also referring to Project Explore as offering limited evidence of efficacy for risk reduction counseling. The CDC does not, however, acknowledge that the ten sessions of Project Explore reduced HIV incidence by 38% over 12 months. Ironically, the control condition in Project Explore was Project Respect client-centered counseling delivered every 6 months for the duration of the study, effectively equalizing the two conditions over the long term.

The CDC's failure to exploit the prevention opportunities offered by HIV testing has not gone unnoticed. Even within the CDC itself, the Division of STD Prevention's 2006 Treatment Guidelines refute the clinical testing guidelines—which actually include public health clinics, community clinics, and primary care settings—the very places where STDs are treated! The 2006 STI Treatment Guidelines state the following about HIV prevention counseling:

> Prevention counseling does not need to be explicitly linked to the HIV-testing process. However, some patients might be more likely to think about HIV and consider their risks when undergoing an HIV test. HIV testing might present an ideal opportunity to provide or arrange for prevention counseling to assist with behavior changes that can reduce risk for acquiring HIV infection. Prevention counseling should be offered and encouraged in all health-care facilities serving patients at high risk and in those (e.g., STD clinics) where information on HIV-risk behaviors is routinely elicited.

Delinking risk reduction counseling from HIV testing has also drawn criticism from leading prevention scientists. David Holtgrave has argued that the preventive value of HIV testing and counseling are intertwined. He notes that HIV testing creates a context for behavior change and counseling provides the tools for change. Holtgrave, a former Director of the Division of HIV/AIDS Prevention at the CDC, draws the following conclusion:

> The CDC has recently expressed concern that quality of counseling typically associated with HIV testing may be substandard in some settings and that it is therefore of little value. However, this means that we have a choice of whether to dismiss counseling or—as many states and localities have done contractually and in program guidelines—to raise its quality to the standard of client-centered counseling, which, according to the CDC, is effective, efficient, and practical in clinical settings. Aspiring to a consistent, client-centered standard of counseling is to be preferred. To do less could be construed as a negligent or harmful act, because withholding an intervention that can reduce incident STDs by 20–30% appears to violate a basic principle of biomedical ethics.
>
> The question of who in the health care system can help us meet client-centered counseling standards, particularly if clinicians do not have the time must be explored. We need to be creative. Non-clinicians in the health care system could provide such counseling. Also, there are opportunities for community-based organizations to have much more active roles

in counseling and testing, perhaps even in partnership with clinic-based health care professionals to ensure the availability of client-centered counseling and testing. In some respects, these agencies may be in a better position than clinicians, who may be too busy or too inexperienced in behavioral counseling, to develop and deliver counseling services at a client-centered standard [96].

The kind of creative thinking that Holtgrave mentions will come from clinical service providers. In Arizona, for example, the Rio Community Health Center developed innovative patient support services that deliver a broad range of evidence-based prevention programs that are integrated with clinical care [97]. These services are not seen as an added burden but rather as part of usual care. In South Africa, STI clinics with significant patient loads under extremely limited resources utilize specialized counselors to deliver HIV testing and counseling. I know from personal experience that South Africans receive counseling with testing that is in keeping with Project Respect's client-centered approach. Thus, delivering risk reduction counseling with HIV testing can occur when prevention policy makers are committed to prevention.

## New Testing Technologies

Advances in HIV testing technologies have expanded services beyond traditional care settings. Rapid HIV tests deliver results in as little as 10 min. People no longer fall through the cracks between collecting a blood specimen and delivering test results. Rapid tests can be performed on saliva samples, making the test quick, non-invasive, and free of biohazards. Noninvasive rapid HIV tests open the door to point of contact HIV testing; bringing testing to emergency rooms, night clubs, festivals, bath houses, and street corners. The advent of rapid HIV tests raised immediate questions about whether effective risk reduction counseling could be delivered with results received within minutes.

To answer this question the CDC conducted Project Respect-2. The aim of this study was to test whether the potent effects of counseling and testing observed in Project Respect could be replicated in the rapid test context. The CDC's Carol Metcalf and Tom Peterman headed up the trial [98]. They randomized patients in US STI clinics to either receive standard 2-week or rapid testing and counseling. The standard condition was essentially the same intervention protocol delivered in the Project Respect study, consisting of pretest counseling, specimen collection, a waiting period, test result notification, and 20-min of client-centered counseling. The rapid testing condition also delivered pretest counseling, but the notification and counseling results were delivered in less than an hour. The counseling content was essentially the same for the two groups, with only slight modifications to meet the formatting of rapid testing. In both conditions, the counseling was personalized and focused on developing a risk reduction plan. Achieving one goal of rapid testing, all of the patients in the rapid testing and counseling condition received risk reduction counseling, whereas only 69% of patients in the 2-week standard condition received their results and posttest counseling.

Results showed that after 1 year of follow-up there was little difference between conditions for incidence of new STI; between 17 and 19% of participants were diagnosed with a new STI, higher than in the original Project Respect, which demonstrated 12% incidence. There was also some evidence that rapid test counseling may be slightly less effective in reducing risk than the standard test. In particular, they found rapid testing and counseling less effective for men than standard testing and counseling, but not so for women. Nevertheless, Project Respect-2 showed equivalent risk reduction outcomes for conducting standard or rapid testing with HIV risk reduction counseling.

Rapid tests have also opened the door to home testing. In 1996 the FDA approved home HIV testing. However, these tests were not truly conducted at home in the same way as performing an early pregnancy test. Rather, individuals purchased a home HIV test kit, collected a drop of fingertip blood and mailed it to the home test company for analysis. Results were delivered a couple weeks later in a phone counseling session for people who tested HIV positive and in an audio message for those who tested HIV negative. Today, HIV tests have been approved for over the counter sale, bringing the entire testing process into the home without any counseling. Home testing has the advantages of privacy, anonymity, low cost, and convenience. Consistent with the CDC's standards for HIV testing, counseling is simply not a consideration.

Home tests may also be used as an impromptu prevention strategy by bringing the test into the context of sexual decision-making. The test can be used to determine whether partners need to use condoms. Individuals who select sex partners based on their perceived or believed HIV status (serosorting) may be interested in this strategy. Ana Ventuneac and Alex Carballo-Dieguez examined whether using home tests to screen sex partners may reduce HIV risks. Mathematical modeling found that in places of higher HIV prevalence, home testing could lower the risk for HIV infection even when considering the uncertainty of unprotected sex during acute infection when the results can be false negative. As population HIV incidence increases, and therefore so too does the likelihood of a partner being acutely infected, the impact of home testing for screening sex partners decreases. Thus, when compared with inconsistent condom use, home testing in high-prevalence communities can reduce risks, but the converse is true in places with high-HIV incidence. Home screening sex partners can actually increase risks for HIV infection because testing will replace condoms in a context where users just won't know the epidemiological dynamics in their community.

A thorn in the side of HIV testing is the period between infection and immune response, a time when antibody tests are vulnerable to false-negative results. It is also during this time when newly infected persons are highly infectious and likely engaging in high-risk behaviors. Although early discussions of acute infection suggested that a large proportion of HIV transmission events occur during these few weeks, those ideas have not been supported by research. However, there is no question that individuals who are told they are HIV negative but are actually acutely infected have the potential to infect multiple partners.

A public health approach to acute infection involves reanalyzing blood samples that have tested HIV antibody negative to determine whether the test was conducted during the window period before immune response. Specimens collected as part of routine screening are subjected to an algorithm that tests and retests the specimens using sensitive and less-sensitive HIV testing and RNA detection procedures. Positive results signal a systematic partitioning of the specimen pool until, ultimately, the positive case is detected. What follows is a visit from a public health worker to the infected person. Mike Cohen and his colleagues at the University of North Carolina demonstrated the potential impact of public health detection of acute HIV infection [99]. In a study of 109,250 persons at risk for HIV infection who had been tested, there were 606 HIV-positive results. Of those, 107 did not test HIV antibody positive and were identified with the use of sensitive–less-sensitive enzyme immunoassays. In addition, 23 persons were found acutely infected only with the use of RNA testing. Although a small number of positive persons were detected, the number of new infections potentially averted could be enormous given that these highly infectious individuals thought that they were uninfected.

An alternative approach to detecting acute infection relies on clinical care. In this case providers are trained to conduct risk assessments with patients presenting with symptoms of acute viral infection. The basis for a clinical approach to detecting acute infection lies in assuming that some number of people newly infected with HIV will seek clinical services for fever, swollen lymph glands, loss of appetite, fatigue, headache, malaise, and rash that can occur within the first few weeks of infection. Lisa Hightow-Weidman at the University of North Carolina found that 75% of persons with acute HIV infection experience symptoms consistent with acute retroviral syndrome [100]. Among those with symptoms, 83% sought medical care but only 15% were appropriately diagnosed at their initial medical visit. Recognizing the symptoms as potentially acute HIV infection can trigger a risk assessment and HIV testing. Current HIV tests that combine antibody and antigen assays improve the sensitivity and specificity of detecting acute infection.

## Lessons (Hopefully) Learned

Recognizing that condoms, needles, and antibody tests are biomedical technologies that have morphed into behavioral interventions provides a history to consider when scaling-up TasP. It is impossible to know how many infections have been averted by these early HIV prevention technologies. Unfortunately, their full prevention potential has never been realized. Let's consider some challenges and barriers that can serve as lessons to learn as we scale-up TasP.

### *Biomedical Technologies Morph into Behavioral Interventions*

All technology ultimately depends on humans for use. In public health, consider vaccines. An efficacious vaccine is useless without access, acceptance, and uptake. The H1N1 flu vaccine in 2009 offers one example. Coverage in the US and Europe was far lower than needed to achieve community-level protection. Confusing communications, misinformation, and public perceptions kept H1N1 vaccine acceptance and uptake low. The same can be said for the scale-up of human papillomavirus (HPV) vaccination, which is safe and nearly 100% effective. In 2010 the CDC reported that only 25% of adolescents 13–17 years old received at least one dose of the vaccine and only 11% reported receiving all three recommended doses. Condoms, needles, HIV testing, and now HIV treatments will only be as effective in practice as their social, cultural, and behavioral dimensions allow. Planning the implementation of TasP should look back on successes and failures of preceding biomedical prevention technologies.

## Shifting Prevention Away from Condoms Toward TasP Will Increase STI Risks

Offering any alternative will reduce condom use. People want to feel safe and they do not want to use condoms. TasP offers this alternative. It is foolish to think that a man who undergoes circumcision to reduce his risk for HIV will continue to use condoms at the same rate he had before he was circumcised. Risk compensation is not an aberration; it is a consequence of human decision-making. When it comes to TasP, contracting an STI increases infectiousness, countering the protective mechanism of TasP. Suggesting that people should continue to use condoms when employing TasP is a doomed message given that the motivation behind TasP is to do away with condoms. To succeed, TasP must include a routinized and aggressive approach to screening and treating STI.

## Medication Adherence Will Be Different for Prevention than It Is for Therapeutics

Asymptomatic patients will not experience overt benefits of treatment. The long-term benefits of early treatment are preventive, and will therefore face the same challenges as other forms of preventive health care. Successful prevention means that something does not happen. We must be better at communicating the expected outcomes from the preventive use of treatments. We already tell patients that if they lapse in their use of antiretroviral medications they run the risk of treatment resistance. This same mindset needs to be part of TasP.

## Social Support Will Bolster the Impact of TasP

A key to the success of TasP will be engagement and retention to care. Supportive networks have proven effective in bolstering prevention with injection drug users, men who have sex with men, and women. There are now established social network methodologies that should be exploited when implementing TasP. Jeff Kelly at the Medical College of Wisconsin, a pioneer in network driven prevention interventions [101–103], is working toward adapting his successful models for treatment engagement and retention. Carl Latkin at Johns Hopkins University is also adapting his network-level interventions for people living with HIV/AIDS. These approaches will be important to the long-term success of TasP.

## TasP Should Not Be Linked to HIV Testing

HIV testing has an identity problem. Testing had been an instrument of prevention, but now testing is solely a diagnostic tool. Connecting TasP to testing in a so-called "test and treat" strategy may place it in politically charged currents that could doom treatments to the same prevention fate as client centered counseling.

## Stigma Remains a Significant Barrier to Care and Will Undermine TasP

There is a socio-cultural AIDS epidemic that runs in parallel to the epidemics of HIV and AIDS. Stephen Morin of the University of California at San Francisco in 1988 first set forth this concept of parallel epidemics [104]. Morin described "the social, cultural, economic, and political reaction to the HIV and AIDS epidemics." He observed, "This third epidemic of reaction, which is just beginning, is as much a part of the pathology of AIDS as the virus itself." Despite our long knowing that AIDS stigma degrades all of our efforts to prevent, test, and treat HIV there is a virtual dearth of stigma interventions. Most AIDS stigma research still relies on the work of Erving Goffman from 1963. Our failure to attract stigma researchers into the field has created a vacuum of knowledge on what could be the single most important social aspect of AIDS.

## A Harm Reduction Perspective Should Frame TasP

We cannot expect 100% protection from any prevention technology, including TasP. If we lead people to believe that TasP is any more protective than it can be, we will have set TasP up to fail. People who use condoms half the time are told that they are not protected. This absolutist message has undermined prevention. If you miss taking the pill, should you just as well consider not using TasP at all? Communicating partial protection is critical, and yet how best to do so is unknown.

# Chapter 3
# The TasP Revolution

*Now we know beyond a doubt: If we take a comprehensive view of our approach to the pandemic, treatment doesn't take away from prevention. It adds to it. So let's end the old debate over treatment versus prevention and embrace treatment as prevention.*

*Secretary of State Hillary Rodham Clinton, Washington, DC, November 7, 2011*

Antiretroviral therapies are the great success in the story of AIDS. There are now several classes of medications to disrupt every point of HIV's replication cycle. When used in combinations, these medications impede the virus' ability to infect immune cells. Treatment has improved the health and extended the lives of millions of people.

The potential for these potent drugs to also prevent HIV transmission is not a new idea. Even in the late 1980s it was known that AZT accumulated at therapeutic levels in the genital tract. But it was not until 1994 when the true potential for treatment to prevent HIV transmission was realized. The AIDS Clinical Trial Group protocol 076 demonstrated that treating HIV-infected pregnant women with AZT significantly reduced the risk of infecting newborns [105]. Heralded as what remains the single greatest breakthrough in HIV prevention, the use of antiretroviral therapies during labor and delivery has saved countless children from HIV infection. The success of treatment in preventing perinatal HIV transmission also forms the basis for exploiting the potential for treatments to prevent the sexual transmission of HIV.

One driving force behind the enthusiasm for TasP is that it uses an available and proven strategy against HIV. With treatments showing remarkable clinical efficacy for people living with HIV, interest in TasP grew greater with every failed vaccine and microbicide. Failure to scale-up effective behavioral interventions also left a vacuum for prevention interventions. Just as Roger Tatoud's model discussed earlier suggests that the pressure for an effective prevention technology escalated as attempts fell flat. Reductions in the cost of treatments also make scaling-up TasP economically feasible, at least in resource-rich countries. Treatments have also become less toxic, better tolerated, and available with simpler dosing. Finally, mathematical models have forecasted the potential for significant impacts of TasP on HIV in developing countries. Even prior to a solid empirical foundation, mathematical models of TasP got the attention of policy makers, pushing the research agenda forward.

S.C. Kalichman, *HIV Treatments as Prevention (TasP):*
*Primer for Behavior-Based Implementation*, SpringerBriefs in Public Health,
DOI 10.1007/978-1-4614-5119-8_3, © Seth C. Kalichman 2013

In addition to its promise, TasP also poses great challenges. The National AIDS Trust Panel in the UK raised several questions about the potential use of TasP [106]. First there are the realities of scaling-up HIV testing, which many see as a precondition for impactful TasP. HIV testing, however, remains low in many high-risk populations. There are also serious questions about just how often individuals who remain at high risk can and should be tested. There are also challenges to TasP presented by acute HIV infection and the potential for persons to falsely test HIV negative in the acute infection stages. Long-term treatment adherence also poses a serious obstacle to TasP. Failure to adhere to medication regimens allows HIV to replicate, undermining the entire strategy. With treatment failure comes risks for developing treatment-resistant strains of virus, which can be transmitted. Even under optimal adherence, viral suppression is not always durable in the long run. Also, viral suppression in blood plasma does not necessarily mean that HIV is suppressed in the genital compartment. There are also concerns about the impact of treatment perceptions and beliefs on sexual and drug use behaviors. The degree to which individuals reduce their condom use and increase risk behaviors will undoubtedly undermine the potential for TasP to prevent infections. To fulfill its promise as a revolutionary prevention strategy, implementing TasP will require solutions beyond the prescription pad.

## The Infectivity Triad

The spread of HIV fundamentally depends on infectivity—the average probability of transmission from an infected host to an uninfected person. Infectivity is primarily determined by three factors: (a) the infectiousness of the infected person, (b) the susceptibility of those exposed to an infected person, and (c) the transmission acts they practice. Prevention strategies aim to impede these spheres of infectivity just as antiretrovirals target HIV's replication cycle (see Fig. 3.1). Infectivity is typically considered in the context of specific behaviors. For example, University of California researcher Nancy Padian was among the first to document HIV transmissibility in heterosexual couples [107]. In her study of HIV serodiscordant couples Padian showed that HIV transmission could be a relatively rare event. She estimated that the infectivity of vaginal intercourse in these couples was around 1 in 1,000. This lower-bound estimate occurred in the context of stable couples where HIV infection had been diagnosed and discussed. Couples were also counseled in strategies for reducing transmission risks, were closely monitored, and were treated for other STI.

Depending on the relative mix of factors, risks for HIV transmission are far greater than 1 in 1,000. The infectivity triad drives sexually transmitted HIV infection [108]. These three factors—infectiousness, susceptibility, and behavior—are the key to HIV transmission and therefore HIV prevention.

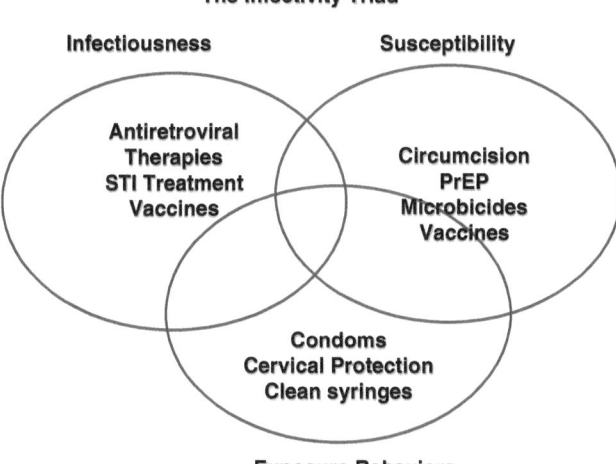

**Fig. 3.1** The HIV Infectivity Triad: source infectiousness, partner susceptibility, and transmission risk behaviors

## *Source Infectiousness*

Concentrations of HIV in blood, semen, and vaginal secretions of infected persons change over the course of HIV infection. People are most infectious soon after they are infected and again nearer to the end stages of AIDS. HIV concentrations in blood and genital secretions peak in the earliest days of infection. During acute infection, the virus is taking hold of the immune system by rapidly replicating and depleting entire populations of immune cells. Infected persons are far more infectious during these early days of the disease than during the subsequent years of chronic infection. As many as half of HIV infections among men who have sex with men in the USA are thought to occur during acute infection [109]. Couples studied in Rakai, Uganda also illustrate the higher risk for HIV transmission during both the acute and late stages of HIV infection. Figure 3.2 shows the results of the Rakai cohort study, which found the highest rates of infections occur in the first and final months of HIV infection [110, 111]. These rates of infections were most obviously driven by HIV viral loads in the infected partners. There were no HIV transmission events when the HIV-positive partner had viral loads under 3,500 copies/ml. Furthermore, half of all infections occurred when the infected partners' viral load exceeded 35,000 copies/ml. The results showed a dose–response relationship, with greater rates of infection incrementally increasing with higher viral loads.

In addition to stage of disease, sexual infectiousness depends on the type/subtype of the virus and its concentration in semen and vaginal fluids. Anything that increases the concentration of HIV in the genital tract will increase infectiousness. Although HIV is harbored in immune cells, which may play important roles in HIV

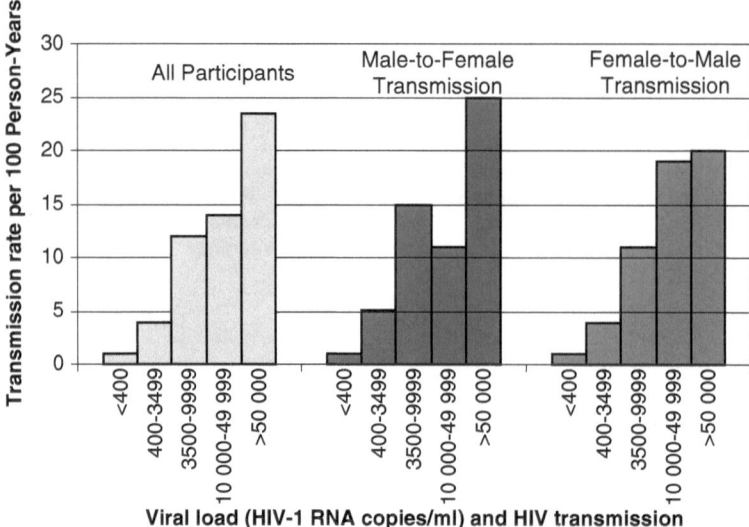

**Fig. 3.2** Associations between HIV viral load and sexual HIV transmission in Rakai Uganda (Wawer et al. [110], used with permission)

transmission, there is now evidence that it is the amount of free virus in blood and genital fluids that ultimately results in most HIV infections. David Butler and Susan Little at the University of California at San Diego genetically analyzed virus detected in men who had recently been infected with HIV and found that the isolates in blood plasma of newly infected men were closely related to the free virus, rather than virus harbored in immune cells. These results showed the primacy of free virus in HIV transmission events. Additional research shows that the amount of virus in semen and vaginal fluids predicts HIV transmission, even when HIV concentrations in blood plasma are statistically controlled. In other words, people who believe they are less infectious based on their having an undetectable blood plasma viral load may very well be far more infectious than they can possibly know. Because effective combinations of antiretroviral medications suppress HIV replication, HIV treatments impact infectiousness. This basic fact is at the core of the logic behind TasP. However, anything that interrupts HIV suppression, such as medication nonadherence or the development of drug-resistant strains of HIV, will conversely increase infectiousness.

Another critical factor in determining the amount of free virus in semen and vaginal fluids is the sexual health of the HIV-infected person. Co-occurring STI cause HIV concentrations to spike in semen and vaginal fluids and thereby increasing infectiousness. Local inflammation of the penile and vaginal mucous membranes stimulates and activates HIV replication, shedding virus and therefore increasing infectiousness. In their review of factors influencing the infectiousness of people living with HIV, Jared Baeten and Julie Overbaugh of the University of Washington reported that genital ulcers increase male-to-female HIV transmission between 10- and 50-fold and female-to-male transmission by 50- to 300-fold. Genital ulcers are especially critical to increasing HIV concentrations in the genital tract. Mike Cohen illustrated how co-occurring STI change the playing field of HIV transmission [112]. What is typically considered the less infectious chronic stage of HIV disease is actually highly infectious when a person is coinfected with another STI. Each incident STI in an HIV-infected person spikes viral shedding in the genital tract, essentially recreating infectiousness that rival acute infection. Similar effects of STI and vaginal inflammation on viral shedding have also been observed, although the effects of anal STI on HIV concentrations in the rectum are less clear.

## Host Susceptibility

People who are sexually exposed to HIV also vary in their risk for infection. Susceptibility to HIV is the product of multiple transmission cofactors. HIV concentrations are generally greater in blood than in semen and vaginal fluids, making any sexual act that involves blood exposure higher risk. For example, men who have sex with an HIV-infected woman during menstruation are more than three times as likely to have HIV infection compared to men who do not engage in sex during menses [113, 114]. It has long been known that sexual exposure to blood increases risks for HIV transmission. For instance, rectal bleeding is a known independent risk factor for HIV transmission during anal sex, increasing risks for HIV several times over. The same is true for vaginal intercourse, where coital bleeding can increase the risk of HIV transmission by more than fourfold [108]. In her heterosexual couples research Nancy Padian observed only one case of female-to-male HIV transmission and that particular couple had repeated instances of vaginal and penile bleeding during intercourse.

Sexual exposure to blood may be one of the most overlooked cofactors in HIV epidemics. Research conducted in a South African township found that 31% of men and 26% of women reported having engaged in sexual intercourse that involved genital bleeding; nearly one in five had done so in the previous 3 months. Three out of four of the times, bleeding was attributed to menses, possibly practiced for contraception [114]. Sex during menses exposes men to higher concentrations of HIV when his partner is HIV infected. Also, vaginal and cervical changes that occur during menses likely increase the HIV susceptibility of uninfected women. In a study conducted in a South African STI clinic, reporting recent sexual bleeding was the single best predictor of a patient becoming HIV infected over the course of a year [115]. Penile, vaginal, and anal cuts and abrasions are also likely sources of sexual bleeding, as are common STI symptoms such as blisters and ulcers.

Beyond coital bleeding, STI increase HIV susceptibility by affording a portal of entry to the blood stream. Even worse, immune cells migrate to the site of local genital infections. Activated to fight initial infection, immune cells express many of the co-receptors that are needed for HIV to bond, enter, and infect cells. When STI are factored into the infectivity equation, we are far from the lower-bound estimate

1 in 1,000 vaginal intercourse occasions. Infectivity for a person with a genital ulcer disease is more than 30 in 1,000 vaginal intercourse occasions and 55 in 1,000 when all STIs are considered. By comparison, infectivity of vaginal intercourse is far less affected by the stage of HIV disease; acute stage infectivity is 5 in 1,000 and late stage infectivity 3 in 1,000 [116].

Also contributing to HIV transmission risks is the concentration of infectable cells exposed to HIV. The virus attaches and enters cells that express specific surface receptors. Only a subset of immune cells found in genital mucous membranes are actually susceptible to HIV infection. In men, the undersurface of the foreskin is particularly vulnerable. The risk for HIV transmission is therefore much higher for uncircumcised men compared to circumcised men. In fact, the relative HIV risk for uncircumcised men is similar to that of men who have genital ulcer disease—but with increased vulnerability during every unprotected sex act. Susceptibility to HIV is also influenced by the ecology of infectable cells. As an enveloped rather than an encapsulated virus, HIV is sensitive to its surrounding environment and quite easily destroyed.

## Risk Behaviors

A person can be highly infectious and their partner can be vulnerable to infection, but HIV transmission will only occur during a couple-specific sex acts; primarily anal and vaginal intercourse without condoms. Behaviors that expose the greatest surface area of infectable cells to the highest concentration of HIV are the most risky. Any breach in the skin or mucous membranes will further increase direct exposure of HIV to infectable cells. Reviews of infectivity research have produced detailed accounts of the relative risks of sexual behaviors. Anal intercourse without condoms carries the highest risk for HIV transmission. Although at relatively lower risk than their receptive partners, men who engage in penile-vaginal or penile-anal intercourse as the insertive partner are also at high risk for HIV infection, especially when their foreskin is intact or when they have an ulcer or some other portal of entry.

Anal sex is the riskiest sexual behavior for HIV transmission because the rectum has an abundance of blood vessels, high concentrations of infectable immune cells, and the potential for intercourse-related trauma. HIV transmission risks to the receptive anal sex partner are several times higher than risks to the insertive partner. Risks accumulate over the course of a relationship, bringing infectivity to as high as 40 in 1,000 acts per partner [116, 117]. Risks of anal sex do not vary for men or women. The relative risks for HIV transmission during vaginal intercourse, for both men and women, are lower than anal intercourse.

Among gay and bisexual men, anal intercourse without condoms is practiced far less now than before the advent of AIDS. The first HIV risk behavioral surveys with gay men were conducted by Tom Coates and Ron Stall in San Francisco who observed reductions in numbers of male sex partners, anal intercourse, and oral intercourse between late 1984 to early 1985 [118, 119]. Research also found that rectal gonorrhea in gay men declined sharply between 1983 and 1984 [119]. Most studies conducted since 1985 have found that one-third of men who have sex with men report unprotected anal sex in some recent time frame. In terms of heterosexuals, rates of anal sex vary but are never as high as vaginal intercourse. Six percent of the US population reports having ever engaged in anal sex in heterosexual relationships, with higher rates among adolescents (16%) [120, 121]. In South African STI clinics, only 10% of patients report engaging in anal sex. The highest rates of anal sex often occur among female sex workers, which can be as high as 40% [122]. Clearly, risks for HIV infection are highest among persons who engage in anal intercourse, especially in high-HIV prevalence places. Nevertheless, there is no evidence that anal intercourse is practiced by sufficient numbers of heterosexuals to be a primary driver of HIV transmission in generalized epidemics [123].

In contrast to anal and vaginal intercourse, oral sex in any form or variation can only be considered lower risk for HIV transmission. However, it seems that oral sex cannot be considered "no risk." There are people who say that they were infected with HIV by performing fellatio and there is no reason to doubt them. These cases are relatively rare and occur in a context where unprotected anal sex is at least 35 times more risky for HIV transmission than engaging in oral sex with a known HIV-positive sex positive partner.

Oral sex is the least understood of sexual risk behaviors for HIV infection and our failure to provide clear evidence-based messages about the relative risks and safety of oral sex is apparent. This uncertainty is the source of considerable anxiety, especially for people with HIV-positive partners and people living in places of high-HIV prevalence. A study of men attending a Gay Pride event in Atlanta found that one in three men expressed feeling anxious about their risks for HIV from practicing oral sex. Men who were anxious about the risks of oral sex also engaged in more oral sex behaviors. In that study, one in five men who were anxious about the risks used a condom the last time they engaged in oral sex, compared to only 6% of men who were not anxious about oral sex risks. The belief that oral sex is safe, or even safer, can lead people to switch from anal or vaginal sex to oral sex. A South African researcher once told me that he found teenagers engaging in more oral sex and less vaginal intercourse, saying that they had figured out the relative risks for themselves. Given the current state of epidemiological research, it is difficult to argue against switching from anal or vaginal intercourse to oral sex as a protective behavior.

## Why Treating HIV Can Prevent Infections

The evidence could not be more compelling; antiretroviral therapies reduce infectiousness in people living with HIV and can prevent HIV transmission. That HIV transmission is linked to the amount of virus in blood plasma was first observed in people who were yet not treated.

The association between blood plasma viral load and sexual transmission of HIV is not, however, the result of a one-to-one correspondence between blood and genital secretion viral loads. In fact, the relationship between HIV in the peripheral circulatory system and the genital compartment is impacted by several factors. Characteristics of the Rakai Cohort discussed earlier may misrepresent the concordance of blood plasma virus and sexual transmission. First there is selection bias. Cohort studies of serodiscordant couples have disclosed their HIV status and have repeatedly undergone HIV testing. Couples who volunteer for research may be motivated to avoid HIV transmission. These couples may also be more stable and less likely to have outside partners than the general population. For example, in the soon to be discussed definitive clinical trial testing TasP, more than 95% of the couples did not report any outside sex partners and less than 5% had an STI at the baseline assessment. Research protocols require repeat HIV testing and risk reduction counseling. In terms of infectiousness, the couples are tested and treated at least semiannually for STI. Thus, serodiscordant couples in research may be far from representative of couples in the real world.

## Beyond Rakai

Observational research conducted under a variety of conditions with diverse populations has mostly supported the Rakai findings. Research in Taiwan, for example, observed no HIV infections in serodiscordant couples when the infected partners had viral loads lower than 1,050 copies/ml [124]. Another study conducted by Baeten and colleagues found a strikingly similar pattern of viral load in relation to HIV transmission, but in this case it was genital tract viral load [125] (see Fig. 3.3a, b). Concentrations of HIV in genital fluids being directly related to HIV transmission risk are not surprising. What is surprising is that genital fluid HIV in relation to transmission risk looks so similar to blood and transmission risk.

The observed associations between viral load and HIV transmission risks in serodiscordant couples logically leads one to consider the potential impact of suppressing HIV to reduce infectiousness. Even before the advent of combination therapies, researchers observed 15% fewer HIV infections in women whose male sex partners were being treated with AZT [126]. Armed with potent combinations of antiretroviral medications bring even greater potential for prevention. In a longitudinal cohort study, Donnel and colleagues at the University of Washington observed only one HIV infection among the 349 couples in which the infected partner had initiated treatment. In contrast, there were 102 HIV infections observed among the 3,032 couples with untreated HIV-positive partners. A review of studies investigating the effects of HIV treatment on transmission did not find a single case of HIV transmission in heterosexual couples when the infected partner was being treated and had a blood plasma viral load under 400 copies/ml [127]. A study conducted in Spain found that HIV infections declined from 10 to 1.9% in relation to increased access to ART [128]. Declining rates of HIV infections have also been observed in relation to increased access to antiretroviral therapies in Taiwan and Denmark [129, 130].

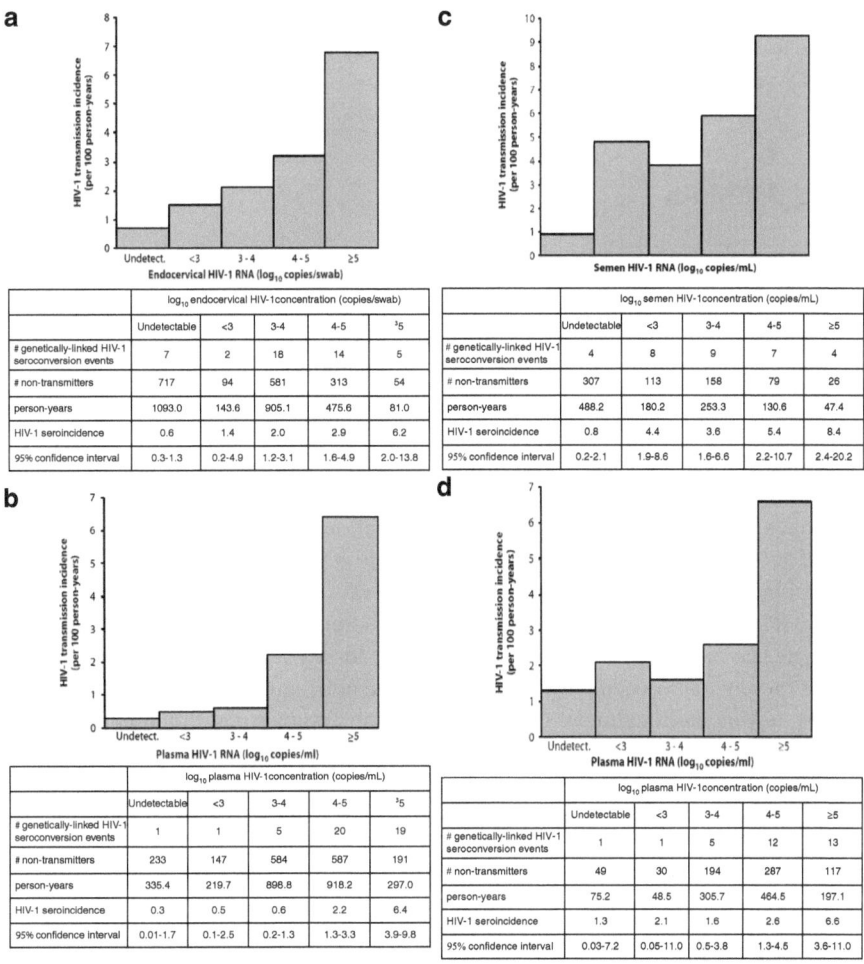

**Fig. 3.3** Step-wise association between genital and plasma HIV RNA quantity and HIV transmission risk. (**a**) and (**b**) Female-to-male transmission showing HIV concentrations in endocervical fluids and plasma, (**c**) and (**d**) male-to-female transmission showing HIV conentrations in semen and plasma (Baeten et al. [125] used with permission)

The impact of treatment on HIV transmission observed at the individual level is not easily extrapolated to populations. Wealthy countries, for example, have relatively unrestricted access to treatment and yet HIV infections either remain stable or continue to rise. Men who have sex with men in Sydney, where antiretrovirals are widely available, demonstrate the same levels of new HIV infections observed since the early 1990s [131]. Major cities in the USA that have access to treatment have not seen reductions in HIV incidence. The lack of impact from treatment on population-level HIV infections does not mean that treatments cannot prevent infections. It is likely that treatment delivered in care does not mimic the attention, monitoring, adherence support, risk reduction counseling, and STI services provided in research.

We assume that the impact observed in serodiscordant couples studies results from treatment alone, when in fact a plethora of interventions are delivered in research that may very well carry the day.

## Doing the Math

Mathematical models can bridge the gap between research and what may occur in the real world. Models are also capable of testing the potential impact of interventions on HIV epidemics under various hypothetical scenarios. As it is often said, mathematical models are only as good as their assumptions. Although the history of AIDS shows that yesterday's mathematical models do not always map onto today's reality, modeling still offers a useful tool for estimating what may be possible.

Models can be formulated to represent best-case and the worst-case scenarios. The most influential optimistic scenario for TasP was represented in a model reported by Reuben Granich at the World Health Organization [132]. This model was indeed framed as "Utopian" in that it assumed a complete scale-up of universal HIV testing and treatment in the poorest countries with the most catastrophic HIV epidemics. The model further assumed universal perfect adherence to achieve 100% viral suppression. The model did not include parameters for the impact of acute infections, partner mixing, or co-occurring STI. Granich and colleagues concluded that universal HIV testing and treatment, under their utopian assumptions, could reduce HIV incidence to less than 1 infection per 1,000 people per year and bring HIV prevalence down to 1% of the population within 50 years. TasP could therefore lead to the end of AIDS. The idea of setting HIV epidemics on a course toward elimination by using tools already in hand rightfully stirred excitement. Carl Dieffenbach and Anthony Fauci of the NIH went as far as to call for implementing a prevention strategy built on HIV testing and treatment [133].

Not surprisingly, mathematical models that use more realistic assumptions have less optimistic forecasts. Realistic models focus on the impact of systematically altering treatment access under population-level conditions. For example, monitoring viral suppression in treated patients is a critical element of TasP. However, information about changes in viral load can impact sexual decisions and behavior. Every study that has examined infectiousness beliefs has found that people who believe they are less infectious engage in higher risk behaviors. Frequency of viral load testing is therefore important. Also important is the degree to which blood plasma viral load actually reflects genital fluid infectiousness. Studies show that when treatment is accompanied by viral load monitoring every 3 months, condom use can be reduced to 9% of sexual occasions while preserving the preventive benefits of treatment [134]. However, scaling-back viral load monitoring to perhaps every 18 months would require at least 70% condom use to sustain the preventive benefits of treatment. Other realistic models have taken acute infection into consideration as well as other factors that influence infectiousness over the course of HIV disease [134]. Curiously few mathematical models include co-occurring STI in their assumptions, and those that do yield the most pessimistic result. The ability of mathematical models to forecast the impact of TasP on the course of HIV epidemics therefore depends on assumptions that may not reflect reality.

We have therefore seen multiple lines of evidence make a strong case in support of TasP. Biological plausibility is shown when treatments effectively prevent HIV transmission from mothers to newborns. Studies of HIV serodiscordant couples also demonstrate the biological plausibility of TasP by showing a reliable association between viral load in blood plasma and HIV transmission. Observational studies of couples receiving treatment further shows that partners who are treated are less likely to transmit HIV. Finally, mathematical models add support by demonstrating the potential impact of treatment on epidemiologic estimates under various assumptions. Despite a compelling case from converging lines of evidence, there is nothing like a randomized clinical trial to rule out alterative explanations and offer definitive proof for the efficacy of TasP.

## Definitive Proof

The HIV Prevention Trials Network (HPTN) is a large collaborating group of international scientists primarily supported by the NIH. Among the most important studies to come from the HPTN is their randomized clinical trial that tested the efficacy of TasP. The study was HPTN 052; the first randomized clinical trial of using HIV treatment to prevent the sexual transmission of HIV [135, 136]. HPTN 052 was conducted in nine southern African countries and randomly assigned 763 HIV serodiscordant couples to one of two experimental conditions: (a) treating the HIV-infected partner early, when his or her CD4 cell count was between 350 and 500 cells/cc$^3$ or (b) delaying treatment for the infected partner until his or her CD4 count fell below 350 cells/cc$^3$—the conditions under which treatment is typically started. The central question asked in HPTN 052 was whether treatment could prevent sexual transmission to an HIV status-discordant partner [137]. In addition, the investigators recognized the duration of treatment benefits would be critical to understanding the true impact of TasP. The study hypothesized that there would be a 30% reduction in HIV transmission that could be attributed to the early start of treatment. A secondary and also important aim of the trial was to test the potential benefits of early treatment for the health of the HIV-infected partner.

Table 3.1 summarizes the key features and findings of HPTN 052. An interim analysis conducted about halfway through the study found the answer. The interim results were deemed irreversible by the study monitoring committee, which recommended stopping the trial. The committee concluded that initiating therapy early substantially protected HIV uninfected sex partners, with as much as a 96% reduction in risk. HPTN 052 observed 39 new HIV infections. Using genetic testing of the viruses obtained from the couples, the researchers determined that 28 of the 39 infections were genetically linked to the HIV-infected partner in the study. Of those 28 genetically linked infections, only one had occurred from a partner receiving

**Table 3.1**  Summary of major study design features and key findings from HPTN 052 trial

| Study design features | Key findings |
| --- | --- |
| • HIV serodiscordant couples participated in the trial | • 39 new HIV infections occurred through April 2011 |
| • 97% of couples were heterosexual | • The trial was stopped early due to compelling prevention outcomes at interim analysis |
| • Couples were randomized to treatments | • Of the 38 infections, 27 occurred in the delayed treatment arm, and one occurred in immediate treatment arm |
| • Conducted at 13 clinical trial centers in Botswana, Brazil, India, Kenya, Malawi, South Africa, the USA, Thailand, and Zimbabwe | • 17 of the 27 infections in the delayed treatment arm occurred when the infected partner's CD4+ T-cell count was greater than 350 |
| • All couples received routine HIV testing and counseling as well as STI detection and treatment throughout the trial | • Eleven unlinked infections could not be genetically traced to the infected partner, indicating multiple partnerships |
| • Adherence was monitored using pill counts and any indication of nonadherence received intensive intervention | • The median viral load for transmitting partners was 4.91 log copies of viral RNS/ml blood |
| | • There were 105 clinical events—65 in delayed treatment arm and 40 in immediate treatment arm |
| | • There were 23 deaths—13 in delayed treatment arm and 10 in immediate treatment arm |

early treatment, with the other 27 occurring among couples that were in the delayed treatment group. Thus, the first study hypothesis was confirmed; early treatment prevented HIV transmission.

With regard to the second aim of the study, whether early treatment would benefit the HIV-infected partner, that hypothesis was also confirmed. Early treatment slowed HIV disease progression. Of the 105 observed clinical health events related to disease progression 65 (62%) afflicted the delayed treatment group. The potential health benefits of early treatment therefore add to the public health benefits.

It should not go unmentioned that 11 of the 39 HIV infections in HPTN 052 stemmed from outside relationship sex partners. Consistent with this finding are observational studies of serodiscordant couples using similar procedures for linking the genetics of partners' viruses. These studies find between 9% and 13% of HIV infections involve partners outside of an established HIV serodiscordant relationship. If TasP will be aimed primarily at serodiscordant couples, it could fail as much as 25% of the time. This finding points to the need for a broader implantation strategy that extends beyond serodiscordant couples. In addition, behavioral interventions that reduce concurrent sex partners will bolster the impact of TasP. Another factor in scaling-up TasP is adherence. In HPTN 052, adherence was carefully monitored by clinic pill counts. Any indication that adherence was less than optimal triggered intensive interventions. As a direct result of HPTN 052, prevention polices in most countries now focus on treating infected persons. The enthusiasm for TasP expressed by leading prevention scientists and policy makers has signaled a major paradigm shift in HIV prevention. However, some policy makers shifted their paradigm even before HPTN 052, namely the Swiss Health Ministry.

## The Swiss

Research showing that treatment reduces HIV infectiousness is compelling. But does receiving HIV treatment render a person noninfectious? Should patients be told not to worry about infecting their HIV negative sex partners? The Swiss Federal Commission for HIV/AIDS answered yes. Based on research primarily conducted by Swiss scientist Pietro Vernazza, the Swiss Federal Commission issued a statement in 2008 that proclaims HIV-infected persons are noninfectious when the HIV-infected person....

- Is adherent to their antiretroviral drug regimen
- Has a suppressed viral load for at least 6 months
- Is free of STI and other genital tract infections

The Swiss Statement draws directly from Pietro Vernazza's cohort studies of Swiss men showing viral load in semen is perfectly concordant with viral load in blood plasma, when men were adherent, viral suppressed, and free of STI [138–140]. The Swiss Statement concludes that there is no need for concern that HIV can be transmitted when an HIV-infected partner is adherent, viral suppressed, and free of STI. As stated in the opening paragraphs by the Statement "One of the objectives of the Swiss National AIDS Commission (EKAF) is to publish new insights on the infectiousness of HIV-positive people on optimally effective therapy. The EKAF wants to alleviate fears of people living with or without HIV and thus wants to allow part of the 17,000 people living with HIV in Switzerland to have as much as possible a 'normal' sexual life" [141].

The Swiss Statement is unambiguous. Along with the specific circumstances under which a person with HIV should be considered noninfectious, the Statement also offers guidelines to clinicians for counseling their patients in light of the new stance on HIV transmission. Providers are advised to inform patients that they no longer need to worry about infecting others with HIV when the conditions of non-infectiousness are met:

> HIV-infected individuals without additional STD and on effective ART, who are not living in a stable partnership, are being informed by their treating physician about their 'non-infectiousness under effective ART'. This information can have a liberating effect as many studies show that the sexual life of HIV-infected individuals are diminished because of fears of infecting others. In the best interests of people living with HIV physicians will continue to recommend Safer Sex to those people having anonymous or occasional sex encounters to minimise risk of additional STDs. Dependent on the amount of such types of sexual contacts regular controls and tests of additional STDs should be performed. Affected persons should be sensitised to symptoms of STD [141].

Almost immediately upon its release, the Swiss Statement brought strong reactions. Those who recognize that infrequent and selective condom use have become the norm for many serodiscordant couples welcomed the Statement. The personal impact of redefining HIV risk from the perspective of people living with HIV was expressed in numerous commentaries and testimonials. Darien Taylor, who had been living with HIV for more than 20 years at the time the Statement was released, offered the following sentiments on the Canadian HIV advocacy Web site CATIE (http://www.positiveside.ca/e/V10I2/Toc_e.htm).

> For most of us, most of the time, the new information that we have about viral load and other factors affecting HIV transmissibility won't make a huge "operational" difference in the way that we have sex. Given the yet-to-be-answered questions about such things as the link between viral load in blood, semen, vaginal and rectal secretions and the contribution of inflammation and STIs to HIV transmissibility, it is difficult to see this new information as a clear go-ahead to abandon condoms. For now and into the foreseeable future, condoms will continue to be our main way of keeping sex safer.
>
> Serodiscordant couples who are trying to conceive will definitely benefit from the Swiss commission's announcement, which is reassuring about the risk of transmitting HIV through unprotected sex, particularly when the positive partner has an undetectable viral load and when the period of unprotected sex is limited. As well, people with HIV who have an undetectable viral load (and our partners) will no longer need to spend sleepless post-coital nights tossing and turning in worry about when the condom happened to break accidentally during the evening's amorous activities. But for many of us, our sex life will probably look much the same as it has throughout this epidemic. We have become attached to the security of condoms and, strange though it seems, to the freedom that they offer us to safely have several sex partners, if we so choose.

The Swiss Statement was taken seriously and signaled a shift in HIV prevention discourse. POZ Magazine founder Sean Strub who contributed an essay in the Huffington Post offered a thoughtful response to the Statement. He wrote, "Interpreting the Swiss statement as 'permission' to stop using condoms would be a mistake, so too would dismissing it altogether or denying its powerful message of hope." He went on to say, "The Swiss have rightly brought viral load into the risk calculus, revolutionizing the paradigm of HIV prevention, and placing condoms in their proper place, as one tool among many to be utilized to prevent HIV transmission. Failing to embrace the opportunity presented by the Swiss statement—to stimulate community discussion, improve the ability of individuals to accurately assess risk and encourage more research—is irresponsible" [142].

Many public health officials found the Swiss Statement at best premature and at worst reckless. The World Health Organization (WHO) and the Joint United Nations Programme on HIV/AIDS (UNAIDS) issued an immediate response to the Swiss Statement in which they said:

> Following the recent publication of an article on antiretroviral treatment and sexual transmission of HIV in the Swiss medical journal 'Bulletin des médecins suisses', UNAIDS and WHO reiterate the importance of a comprehensive approach to HIV prevention including correct and consistent use of condoms. The article, published by Switzerland's Federal AIDS Commission (La Commission fédérale pour les problèmes liés au Sida), states that seropositive individuals do not risk transmitting HIV to a seronegative partner under the following conditions: The seropositive partner has to have had undetectable HIV in the

blood for at least 6 months, there must be strict adherence to his/her antiretroviral regimen, and he/she must be free of any other sexually transmitted infections. In the article the Commission states that although available medical and biological evidence does not rule out the possibility of HIV transmission they feel that there is nonetheless enough information to support its statement.

To prevent transmission of HIV, UNAIDS and WHO strongly recommend a comprehensive package of HIV prevention approaches, including correct and consistent use of condoms. People living with HIV who are following an effective antiretroviral therapy regimen can achieve undetectable viral loads (the amount of virus in a body fluid such as blood, semen or vaginal secretions) at certain stages of their treatment. Research suggests that when the viral load is undetectable in blood the risk of HIV transmission is significantly reduced.

However, it has not been proven to completely eliminate the risk of transmitting the virus. More research is needed to determine the degree to which the viral load in blood predicts the risk of HIV transmission and to determine the association between the viral load in blood and the viral load in semen and vaginal secretions. Research also needs to consider other related factors that contribute to HIV transmission including comorbidity with other sexually transmitted diseases. UNAIDS and WHO will continue to follow the science of HIV transmission and the effect of antiretroviral treatment on the transmission of HIV.

UNAIDS and WHO underline the importance of effective and proven HIV prevention methods for all people irrespective of their HIV status. In 2005 UNAIDS published a policy position paper on HIV prevention to provide policy guidance on intensifying HIV prevention efforts.

A comprehensive HIV prevention package includes, but is not limited to, delaying sexual debut, mutual fidelity, reduction of the number of sexual partners, avoidance of penetration, safer sex including correct and consistent male and female condom use, and early and effective treatment for sexually transmitted infections [143].

Public health organizations and prevention scientists around the world echoed the WHO/UNAIDS. Going from less infectious to noninfectious was considered too broad a leap based on the evidence at the time. To some degree, the Swiss Statement is vindicated by the results of HPTN 052. The WHO now endorses a public health policy to prioritize treatment for public health benefits. The WHO points to HPTN 052 in shifting toward a policy where treating HIV-positive partners with $\geq 350$ CD4 cells/cc$^3$ in serodiscordant couples is recommended to reduce HIV [143]. The WHO's position reflects a more general movement that calls for all HIV-infected partners in serodiscordant couples with CD4 cell counts between 350 and 500 cells/cc$^3$ to qualify for treatment as a way to curb HIV transmission. Thus, while opposition to the Swiss Statement is tempered by compelling evidence that treatment reduces infectiousness, there are few HIV prevention experts willing to say that an undetectable viral load in blood plasma means that a person is noninfectious.

# How TasP Can Fail

Looking back on the history of HIV prevention, there are many times when hope rather quickly dissipated to disappointment. But unlike failed vaccines, ineffective microbicides, and unused behavioral interventions of the past, we know that TasP can be scaled-up. The compelling evidence for TasP efficacy is complemented by an established and globally scalable delivery system. TasP therefore represents an unprecedented opportunity for HIV prevention.

TasP is built on six fundamental assumptions. First, TasP requires low rates of undetected HIV, especially minimal acute infections, in the target population. Second, and perhaps most obvious, TasP requires medication adherence to fully suppress HIV replication. Third, TasP aims to reduce infectiousness, so it assumes a close association between blood plasma HIV viral load and viral load in genital secretions. A fourth assumption of TasP is that concentrations of HIV in the genital immune compartment remain relatively stable. Fifth, TasP assumes relative stability of sexual behavior. Finally, TasP assumes that individuals remain free of sexually transmitted coinfections. Like the popular block stacking game Jenga, the tower of TasP depends on several interlocking assumptions, violating any of which will cause the entire structure to collapse.

## Acute HIV Infection

The onset of HIV infection is marked by a series of biological events that make it a particularly important time for HIV transmission. HIV begins replicating immediately after infection. The first 7–21 days of infection constitute the eclipse phase, which is characterized by a tremendous amount of viral activity. Viral replication is rampant and mostly unchecked. An early immune response is hampered because the virus is infecting key cells that are responsible for signaling immune protective mechanisms. New virus particles produced in mucosal tissues drain to the lymphatic system. Infected persons will often, but by no means always, experience symptoms of acute viral infection, such as fever, swollen lymph nodes, and perhaps flu-like symptoms. Acute HIV infection can last as long as 10 weeks, with viremia—and therefore infectiousness—peaking at about 4 weeks after the onset of infection.

HIV antibodies are produced during acute infection, with the infected person "seroconverting" from HIV negative to positive. The eclipse phase of acute infection ends as viral RNA and antibodies mount in blood plasma. The challenge that acute infection poses to TasP is simple; people who are highly infectious can go undetected if tested during a period of high-risk behaviors. An estimated 9–17% of HIV transmissions in the USA may occur during acute and recent HIV infection [144]. Because the preventive benefits of treatment depend on detecting and treating HIV infection, failure to detect infected persons when they are seroconverting will undermine TasP.

If TasP can successfully reduce HIV infections there will, of course, ultimately be fewer acute infections. Testing technologies that allow for affordable detection of acute infection will play a key role in that success. HIV tests that detect antigens as well as antibodies are improving our capacity for early detection. Retesting batches of HIV antibody negative blood samples for HIV RNA can also identify infected persons who have falsely tested HIV negative [99]. Clinical interventions that rely on health care providers to recognize symptoms of acute infection are also important in closing the virus positive—antibody negative window.

## Adherence

Nothing could be more obvious than the simple fact that medications only work when people take them. The goal of antiretroviral therapies is the complete suppression of HIV replication. Although medication regimens vary in terms of just how much adherence is needed to achieve viral suppression, most combinations of medications require at least 85% adherence. Minimal levels of adherence needed to sustain viral suppression are not necessarily the same across compartments of the immune system [134]. Viral load can have transient spikes or rebound in the genital tract, even when blood plasma viral load remains undetectable. Studies show that the risk for HIV transmission among persons receiving treatment can be as high as 22% [134].

Another complicating factor is that treatment regimens vary in their penetration of the genital tract. High concentrations of most nucleoside and non-nucleoside reverse transcriptase inhibitors are recovered from the genital tract, whereas protease inhibitors achieve lower drug concentrations in this compartment [137]. Suppression of HIV in the genital tract determines infectiousness in semen and vaginal fluids and therefore the risks posed by vaginal intercourse. However, HIV transmission risks associated with anal intercourse are more closely tied to blood exposures. Because concentrations of protease inhibitors are high in blood, these drugs may play a greater role in reducing infection risks from anal sex. A study of men who have sex with men in Seattle found that HIV RNA was detectable in the anal-rectal mucosa in 49% of men not being treated for HIV, compared with 30% in men who were treated with non-protease inhibitor regimens, and 17% in men who were receiving protease inhibitor-based regimens [137].

Beyond the barriers typically encountered in sustaining adherence, TasP poses unique challenges. Treating people early before they experience symptoms or complications of HIV infection will require different motivation than treating people whose immune system is in decline. People who start treatment later in HIV infection experience the benefits of improved health and quality of life. However, TasP will not necessarily bring any experiences of improved health, and may therefore have intermittent use. Starting and stopping treatment is a strong predictor of developing treatment-resistant virus. Thus, another challenge to long-term adherence posed by TasP is its use in the context of committed relationships. People who accept treatment to prevent infecting their serodiscordant partners will be asked to continue treatment and maintain adherence even if their relationship ends.

## Plasma Viral Load and Sexual Infectiousness

TasP requires monitoring of blood plasma viral load as a standard part of clinical care. Before treatment was also used for prevention, viral load was monitored as an indicator of treatment progress and disease progression. With TasP, concentrations of HIV RNA in blood plasma are used to make inferences about sexual infectiousness. The probability of HIV transmission correlates with concentrations of HIV in the relevant host secretions, whether it is blood in percutaneous transmission and

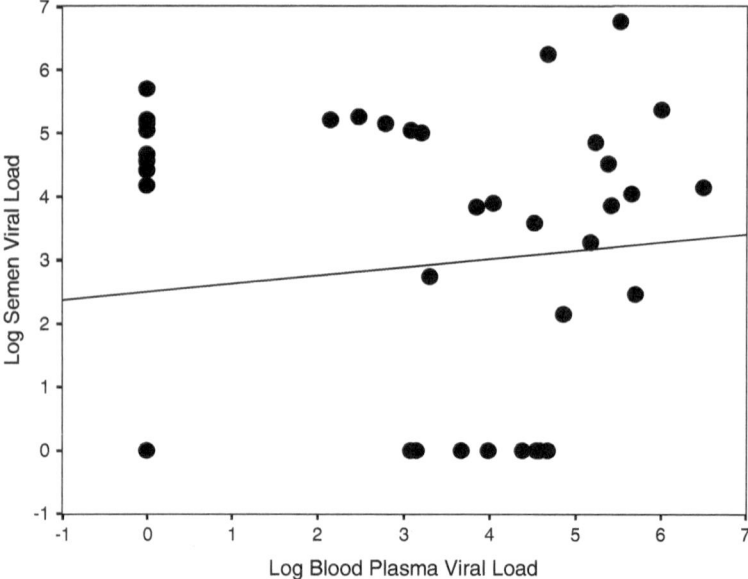

**Fig. 3.4** Scatter plot of HIV viral load in blood plasma and semen of men recruited from multiple sources in Atlanta, GA (Kalichman et al. [148])

mother-to-child transmission, or genital tract fluids in sexual transmission. Changes in viral load can occur quickly. Thus, the more frequent viral load is monitored the more likely changes will be detected, signaling the need for intervention [134].

Sexual infectiousness is determined by genital tract viral load. We have seen that HIV concentrations in genital fluids predict sexually transmitted HIV independent of blood plasma viral load [127]. HIV concentrations in genital secretions also tend to be lower than blood plasma viral load. An estimated 1-log decrease in blood plasma viral load can reflect a 2½-fold reduction in risk for HIV transmission [145]. Thus, in the absence of mitigating factors, a person will likely be less infectious than indicated in their blood plasma.

Nevertheless, a review of 19 studies that tested the association between HIV viral loads in semen and blood plasma found an average correlation of 0.44; knowing the amount of virus in blood plasma accounted for as little as 16% of the variability in HIV in semen [146]. Several factors likely account for this poor association, perhaps most importantly adherence and co-occurring STI. Studies of men who have undetectable blood plasma viral loads, and who are carefully monitored and treated for genital tract coinfections, still find that as many as half periodically have detectable virus in their semen [147].

In a study that my research group conducted with HIV-positive men in Atlanta, we did not find any association between blood plasma and semen viral loads [148]. Figure 3.4 shows the correspondence, or really the lack of any correspondence, between blood plasma and semen viral loads in our study. The correlation was essentially zero. Men who had an undetectable viral load in their blood plasma and were highly infectious in their semen were as common as men who had high viral loads in their blood plasma and low semen viral loads. Failing to find any association between blood plasma and semen viral loads in this study is particularly disturbing because men were recruited from the community. Some men were receiving care and some men were not. Some men were being treated for HIV, others were not. And some men were adherent to treatment while others were not. These men were not part of an ongoing cohort study that would, among other things, routinely monitor and treat STI. These results may therefore be closer to the reality of how blood and semen viral loads correspond.

Studies of viral load concordance in blood and vaginal fluids have found similar magnitudes of association. Research reported by Baeten and colleagues found a 0.56 correlation between blood and vaginal fluid viral loads in women [125]. Cu-Uvin and colleagues observed women who had fully suppressed HIV in their blood plasma [149]. The results showed that 54% of women had detectable virus in their genital tract at least once and 32% had detectable virus in their vaginal fluids while their blood plasma viral load remained undetectable. Viremia in the female genital tract is probably affected by the same factors that can spike viral load in semen, including poor penetration of antiretrovirals in the genital compartment of the immune system, poor treatment adherence, and STI. Gender-specific factors are also important, including changes in HIV concentrations that can occur during pregnancy and various phases of the menstrual cycle [150, 151].

## Beliefs Trump Behavior

Risk compensation occurs as people perceive themselves at lower risk and stop taking protective actions. One thing that makes TasP attractive is that it removes the need to use condoms. There is no reason to expect condom use or other protective actions to remain constant as people continue TasP. However, TasP-related behavioral decision-making is far more complicated than it appears. Whereas condoms interfere with sexual pleasure, they offer a greater certainty of protection than an undetectable viral load. How individuals and couples balance these perceived costs and benefits has not been the subject of research. The impact of risk compensation on TasP is also complex because risk behaviors and infectiousness have different associations with HIV transmission risks. The preventive benefits of TasP can be offset, or even reversed, with increased vulnerability to STI and the development of treatment-resistant HIV in the genital tract [129].

There is compelling evidence that the associations between infectiousness beliefs and sexual risk behaviors are robust. An influential meta-analysis published by Nicole Crepaz and her colleagues at the CDC in 2004 showed a clear relationship between infectiousness beliefs and sexual risk behaviors. The magnitude of the association was sizable and consistent across studies. Again, every study that has

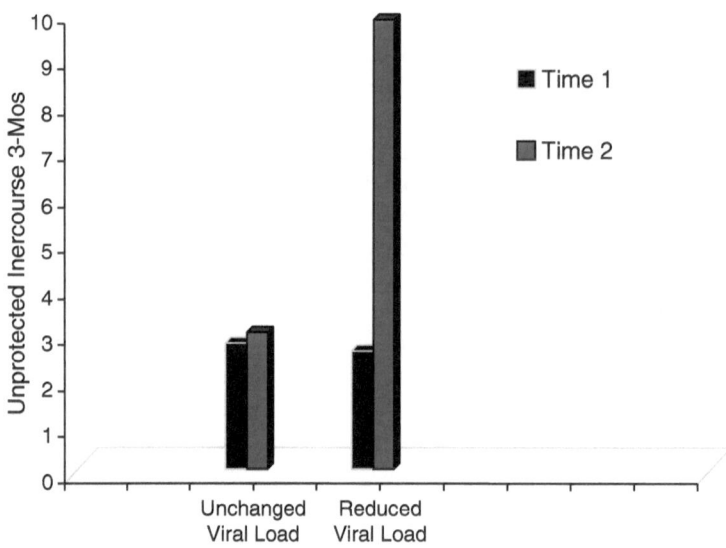

**Fig. 3.5** Impact of changes in HIV viral load on sexual transmission risk behavior in people living with HIV/AIDS (Kalichman et al. [153])

measured infectiousness beliefs has found people who believe they are less infectious when their viral load is undetectable engage in higher risk behaviors. These findings were in contrast to studies that found no associations between treatment and sexual behavior as well as those that examined the relationship between viral load and sexual behavior. Starting treatment and achieving an undetectable viral load in and of itself does not have a consistent influence on behavior. It is the belief that one is less infectious that leads to less condom use and therefore greater unprotected sex.

One study conducted in Atlanta found that HIV-infected individuals who believed they were less infectious when their viral load was undetectable reported substantially more unprotected sex with uninfected sex partners than their counterparts who did not hold these beliefs. However, the relationship varied depending on whether their viral load was undetectable [152]. People who endorsed lower infectiousness beliefs and had undetectable viral loads demonstrated higher risk behavior. This pattern was in contrast to people who did not maintain infectiousness beliefs.

Another study found significant increases in unprotected sexual behaviors when viral load declined from detectable to undetectable [153]. A cohort of 150 men and women that we followed for 8 months found 16 participants who initially had detectable viral loads reversed to having an undetectable viral load. The difference in sexual behavior change between those who had changed to an undetectable viral load was remarkable (see Fig. 3.5). Rates of unprotected sex remained relatively stable for those whose viral load either did not change, or changed from undetectable to detectable. In contrast, those with viral loads that changed from detectable to undetectable demonstrated a dramatic increase in risk behavior. Coinciding with these behavior changes, there were shifts in risk perceptions and infectiousness beliefs. Individuals who went from detectable to undetectable viral load also increased their beliefs that viral load impacts their infectiousness and significantly reduced their concern about infecting their sex partners, despite their increase in sexual risk practices.

Another noteworthy finding comes from the Swiss Cohort Study [154]. Researchers examined the impact of the Swiss Statement itself on risk behavior among men and women and their relationships. There was a clear trend toward increased unprotected sex over time, even before the Statement was released. However, the trend was steeper after the Statement, with increased unprotected sex observed in individuals with stable serodiscordant partners when receiving treatment and their viral load was undetectable. With these increases in unprotected sex come risks for STI and therefore greater infectiousness.

## Sexually Transmitted Coinfections

HIV can replicate in the genital tract even when suppressed in blood. Studies that examine concentrations of HIV in blood and genital fluids show that viral load tends to be lower in genital tract than blood plasma. But this trend is reversed when a person is coinfected with HIV and another STI. Recall our review of studies reporting the association between semen and blood plasma concentrations of HIV RNA found an average correlation of 0.44, with associations ranging between no relationship ($r = 0.07$) and nearly perfect concordance (98%), which only occurred when STI were controlled [146].

HIV concentrations in genital fluids for both men and women are directly associated with the number of leukocytes found in the genital tract. In fact, there is a dose-relationship between leukocytes, a marker for inflammatory disease processes, and HIV viral shedding. Importantly, not all STI equally promote HIV shedding. In general, the greater the inflammatory response to an STI the greater the impact the STI will have on HIV infectiousness. Gonorrhea and Chlamydia are associated with high concentrations of leukocytes in the genital tract, and are therefore related to greater HIV shedding. Bacterial vaginosis also plays a critical role in infectiousness, increasing viral shedding by as much as sixfold [155]. Syphilis, as a blood-borne disease, also increases HIV concentrations in blood plasma, as well as the genital tract. On the other hand, human papillomavirus (HPV) does not significantly impact inflammatory responses in the genital compartment and is not associated with HIV shedding. The STI with greatest impact on HIV shedding are therefore those that produce genital ulcers and urethral/vaginal discharge.

A review of 37 studies of HIV and STI coinfection prevalence found an overall mean STI point prevalence of 15% (SD = 12.4, Median = 12.4) [156]. In southern Africa the average prevalence was 11%, whereas North America demonstrated 16% average prevalence. The most common STI studied was Syphilis, with a median

9.5% prevalence. Also commonly reported were gonorrhea (median prevalence 9.5%), Chlamydia (5%), and Trichamoniasis (18.8%). In most studies, prevalence hovered between 5 and 15%. However, six studies reported STI coinfection prevalence over 30%. Prevalence was greatest at the time of HIV diagnosis, perhaps reflecting the role of STI in HIV transmission. Prevalence of STI among individuals receiving HIV treatment was not appreciably different from untreated persons.

## Implementing TasP

Following the publication of the HPTN 052 trial, there was an immediate ground swell of support for the rapid scale-up of early treatment for people diagnosed with HIV infection. However, some public health advocates raised questions about the potential for drug resistance, risk compensation, long-term use, adherence, patient rights to refuse treatment, structural issues in health service delivery, and justifying the prioritization of treatment for prevention over treatment for disease management. These concerns are legitimate, but seem overshadowed by the health benefits of increased access to treatment and its potential impact on HIV transmission.

It is important to recognize that advancing TasP will only effectively prevent HIV transmission from a subgroup of people living with HIV. David Holtgrave and his colleagues showed that a majority of people in the USA who know that they are HIV infected do not engage in behaviors that risk infecting others, either by not being sexually active or only engaging in sexual activities with HIV-positive (sero-concordant) partners [157]. These individuals will not spread the virus and are not relevant to the scale-up of TasP. Another significant subpopulation of HIV-infected persons are not aware of their HIV status and are therefore not candidates for TasP. Overall, less than 15% of the estimated 1.1 million Americans living with HIV/AIDS are targets for TasP. Holtgrave's model suggests that stemming the tide of HIV transmission will require ramping-up HIV testing and linkage to comprehensive services, especially to the 20% of people with HIV unaware of their status.

Holtgrave and his colleagues have also shown that treating HIV alone will not be sufficient to achieve substantial reductions in HIV infections [157]. In a mathematical model that examined multiple policy scenarios set forth in the US National HIV/AIDS Strategy, they found that the most realistic and cost-efficient means of achieving national prevention goals by 2015 would require investments in expanded HIV detection and diagnostic services as well as prevention services for people living with HIV/AIDS. The most effective and cost-effective policy will therefore scale-up what has been called positive prevention, in addition to increased investments in testing and treating. Positive prevention consists of a family of social and behavioral interventions that have been demonstrated effective in reducing HIV transmission risk behaviors [158]. To succeed, TasP will require integrated approaches that combine antiretrovirals with positive prevention, simultaneously suppressing viral replication, reducing risk compensation, and averting sexually transmitted coinfections.

# Integrating Behavioral Interventions with TasP

Dispensing antiretrovirals alone will not achieve the HIV prevention goals of TasP. The success of TasP requires combining treatment with behavioral interventions to retain patients in care, enhance medication adherence, and aggressively prevent, detect, and treat sexually transmitted coinfections. There are dozens of evidence-based behavioral interventions tested in controlled trials that can be adapted and integrated with TasP. These include sexual risk reduction, injection drug use risk reduction, and medication adherence interventions. The key to success in TasP will be bringing together the optimal combination of behavioral interventions. There are generally two approaches to combining interventions with multiple targeted outcomes. First is an additive approach; stringing together individual interventions to directly impact multiple outcomes. A second approach integrates interventions to target common underlying factors that indirectly impact multiple outcomes. Each approach has been tested with positive results. These interventions have thus far been tested in the USA, with trials underway in Africa [159]. Three particular interventions tested in controlled trials provide viable models that could be immediately integrated with TasP.

## *The Healthy Living Project*

Taking a case management approach, the Healthy Living Project aimed to reduce HIV transmission risks by concentrating on three primary objectives: reducing stress and improving coping; reducing sexual risk practices; and improving antiretroviral medication adherence. Conducted from 2000 to 2002, the trial that tested the Healthy Living intervention is among the largest behavioral intervention trials for people living with HIV/AIDS. A total of 936 HIV-positive men and women in New York, San Francisco, Los Angeles, and Milwaukee participated. Eligibility criteria included reporting at least one unprotected vaginal or anal sexual event with an HIV negative or unknown HIV status partner or non-primary HIV-positive partner in the previous 3 months. The trial randomized participants to the Healthy Living intervention or a control group that received no additional services. Participants were followed for 25 months.

The Healthy Living Intervention was long and intensive. The intervention consisted of 15 90-min one-on-one counseling sessions broken into three modules of five sessions each. The sessions were spread out over 9 months. The first five sessions were conducted weekly, followed by a 3-month break. At month five, the second module of counseling started another five weekly sessions followed by another 3-month break. The final 5-week module began around month 11. The intervention was grounded in Craig Ewart's Social Action Theory, a widely used framework in health behavior interventions [160, 161]. Social Action Theory has a multilevel perspective that takes into account the physical environment, social relationships, mood, and biological conditions. Self-change occurs within the context of these elements through a series of interactive and interdependent processes. Thus, it is essentially a self-regulation theory that takes the social and environmental context into account.

As described in a paper by Cheryl Gore-Felton and the team of investigators, the first five sessions of Healthy Living targeted quality of life, psychological coping, and achieving positive life meaning as a person living with HIV/AIDS [162]. The first session of the coping module began with a discussion between the counselor and participant about perceived strengths and challenges related to health. The counselor conducted a thorough intake evaluation that spanned topics as broad as medical, psychiatric, and substance use histories, stigma and discrimination experiences, social relations, education, and family. The session ended with setting reasonable goals to work on during the remaining sessions. The second and third sessions were developed from coping effectiveness training [163, 164]. The counselor engaged the participant in a series of exercises aimed to identify common stressors and current practices for dealing with stress. Once identified, the stressors were examined for potential coping strategies. In keeping with Coping Effectiveness Training, strategies were defined as emotion or problem focused. The goal of these sessions was to help participants acquire new skills needed to effectively use emotion-focused coping strategies to deal with unchangeable stressors and problem-focused strategies for changeable stressors.

The fourth session carried forward the coping skills to specifically address social support as a means of managing stress. The counselor and participant identified current sources of social support. Members of the participant's personal support network were discussed with an eye toward who can best be relied on for informational, tangible, and emotional support. Strategies concentrated on communication skills to help build positive supportive networks. The fifth and final session of the first module discussed personal successes and remaining challenges in maintaining adaptive coping strategies and positive sources of support. The focus was turned toward realistic goal setting. Of particular importance was a plan for improving coping and support over the following 3 months before the next intervention session.

Three months later the second module commenced, which focused on avoiding sexual and drug use behaviors that increase the risk of HIV transmission. Session 6 of the intervention used the common activity known as a risk continuum, where the participant considered a wide range of sexual behaviors and their potential risks for transmitting HIV. Participants placed behaviors printed on cards on the risk continuum to show how much risk they believed each act confers for HIV transmission. The end result was a powerful visual image that shows only three behaviors at the highest risk end, anal and vaginal intercourse without condoms and sharing injection drug equipment, and numerous behaviors that are either low or no risk for transmitting HIV. This activity served as a springboard to a discussion of the participant's own transmission risk behaviors—essentially framing the next four sessions.

Session 7 picked up from the risk continuum to focus on the seriousness of contracting co-occurring STI. A major part of the session was concerned with the different types of STI and strategies for detecting and avoiding them. Participants learned about condom use and addressed the cultural, relationship, gender, and power influences associated with their own condom use. Self-identified challenges to using condoms were the basis for problem solving exercises to increase condom use. Relationships and other contextual factors were key to this component. The theme of relationships was extended to Session 8, which focused on building communication and sexual negotiation skills. The counselor used modeling and role-plays in well-established assertive communication skills building exercises. Participants set personal goals for negotiating safer sex and safer drug use behaviors.

Session 9 was dedicated to managing more effective HIV status disclosure decisions with sex and drug use partners. Participants identified the circumstances in which they choose to disclose their HIV status and the circumstances when they conceal their status. Stigma, fear, and rejection are typical barriers to disclosure and received special attention in the session. The skills targeted in this session were the identification of personal and environmental factors related to disclosure decisions and increased ability to disclose HIV status. In the final session of the second module, Session 10, the counselor reviewed all of the skills developed thus far and the participant set goals for maintaining safer behaviors while maintaining effective coping and support.

The final intervention module was focused on health services, adherence to health promotion regimens, and negotiating the health care system. Because 25% of the participants in the Healthy Living study were not taking antiretroviral therapies, there were two tracks for this module; one for participants engaged in care and one for those who were not. The primary difference between the tracks was that those who were not engaged in care were encouraged to access medical treatment, as well as develop and follow a self-care plan. Session 11 focused on current health status and understanding health markers—especially CD4 counts and viral load. The discussions included antiretrovirals as well as the use of complementary and alternative medicines. Session 12 was aimed toward medical decision-making. This session used concepts from the earlier sessions on disclosure decision-making applied to this new domain. For example, problem-solving schema were applied to barriers to assertive communication with medical providers.

Session 13 carried on the theme of using already developed skills to improve health. In this case, the connection between social support and adherence. The counselor worked with the participant to identify perceptions of medical or personal health care adherence. Again, problem solving was applied to barriers that reduce health care adherence as well as challenges to obtaining positive sources of social support that influence adherence to health care. The final two sessions of the intervention concentrated on pulling together the skills developed, setting goals, and developing an action plan for long-term success.

The results of Healthy Living study found positive outcomes for both sexual transmission risk reduction and medication adherence. After adjusting for baseline differences on outcome variables between conditions—a significant challenge to the outcome analysis—the results showed that the Healthy Living Intervention had significantly lower transmission risks compared to the control condition at the 15- and 20-month follow-ups, although not at the 5-, 10-, and 25-month follow-ups.

The overall difference was, however, significant [165]. With respect to adherence, significant differences between conditions were observed at the 5- and 15-month follow-ups, which corresponded with the coping and health improvement modules [166]. The outcomes therefore showed an uneven pattern that reflected the proximity of target behaviors to the modules keyed to those behaviors. As an additive model, the findings suggest that behavioral outcomes may not generalize across intervention domains.

## Keeping Healthy and Active with Risk Reduction and Medication Adherence

Although case management services are typically delivered one-on-one, small groups have proven to be effective across multiple domains of health behaviors and have been found cost-effective as well [167, 168]. For people living with HIV, group interventions are particularly accessible in support groups and medication adherence groups. Marcia McDonnell Holstad and Colleen DiIorio at Emory University developed a small group intervention to both improve medication adherence and reduce risks for sexual transmission for women living with HIV. The Keeping Healthy and Active with Risk Reduction and Medication Adherence (KHARMA) intervention was delivered in eight weekly sessions, each lasting between 90 and 120 min and implemented by two trained group facilitators. Groups were conducted in infectious disease clinics in Atlanta. The intervention was guided by the Transtheoretical Model of Behavior Change [169] and relied heavily on techniques adapted from Motivational Enhancement Therapy [170].

The KHARMA intervention focused on eight topics, one each week. The intervention was divided into two major components; first focusing on medication adherence and second on risk reduction behaviors [171]. Table 3.2 summarizes the components and motivational strategies delivered in each session. The first session introduced the group, established ground rules, built rapport, and discussed the goals of the group in the context of lifestyle choices. The next two sessions were focused on medications, treatment goals, adherence, and health. Session 4 was also medication focused, with the group sharing successes and strategies for maintaining adherence. The group shifted its focus in session 5 to sexual risk reduction. Basic risk-related knowledge, condom skills, communication, and sexual negotiation skills were the major areas of attention in sessions 5 and 6. Session 7 was dedicated to HIV status disclosure decision skills. The final group session developed goals and action plans for maintaining medication adherence and safer sexual behaviors.

The KHARMA intervention was tested in a randomized trial that had a time-matched health-behavior comparison condition [172]. A total of 207 women were randomly assigned to one of the two study conditions and followed for 9 months. The results were mixed. In an intent-to-treat analysis, there were no differences between the conditions in electronically monitored medication adherence. However, when examined for intervention exposure, there was evidence for greater adherence among women who had actually attended the intervention sessions. A similar pattern of

**Table 3.2** Content and strategies for the KHARMA intervention (adapted from Holstad et al. [171])

| Session | Content | Strategies |
|---|---|---|
| 1 | Introduction, group guidelines, exploration of lifestyles | Group introductions, icebreaker. Explore day-to-day experiences with medication taking and practicing safer sex RRB. Discuss personal values and how they also fit into one's life. Introduction to goal setting. |
| 2 | ART awareness: the good things and the not so good things | Identify barriers and facilitators for taking ART. Revisit personal values and discuss connections between current medication taking and values. Goal setting. |
| 3 | ART adherence: change and exploring goals | Explore personal motivation for treatment adherence. Problem solving strategies to reduce barriers to adherence. Goal setting. |
| 4 | Sharing successes and treatment strategies | Explore previous successes in lifetime (graduation, etc.); draw from these to enhance medication-taking success. Examine self-confidence to maintain strategies. Explore values and relate to current medication taking behavior. Goal setting. |
| 5 | Risk reduction behavior: knowledge and skills | Discuss "truth or lies" about all risk reduction methods. Male and female condom skill building. Goal setting. |
| 6 | Risk reduction behavior: balance and negotiation | Decisional balance on the pro/cons of using RRB. Explore personal motivation and self-confidence to use RRB consistently. Team consult with role-play safer sex negotiation. Goal setting. |
| 7 | Disclosure of HIV status: to tell or not to tell | Using a case scenario, discuss the good and not so good things about disclosure, and related to sexual behavior. Explore personal self-confidence to disclose and role-play disclosure scenarios. Goal setting. |
| 8 | Summary and termination: putting it all together with goals and values | Safer sex behavior continuum. Identify one's core personal values and link them with current and future medication adherence and use of RRB. Group closure and goodbyes. Certificates of completion. Set long-term goals. |

results was observed for sexual risk behavior, with no differences between groups in the intent-to-treat analysis, but greater sexually protective behaviors among women who attended the intervention sessions. The results were therefore encouraging for those women motivated to attend the groups. Unfortunately, it may be the women who were not motivated to attend the intervention that are of greatest concern.

## In The Mix

In an effort to develop a strategy that would simultaneously improve medication adherence and reduce sexual transmission risks, my research group developed an integrated intervention with two primary outcomes: increased medication adherence and reduced risks for STI. Our approach was to develop a fully integrated model on several dimensions. The content was integrated to address social and

**Conflict Theory of Decision Making**                **Intervention Components**

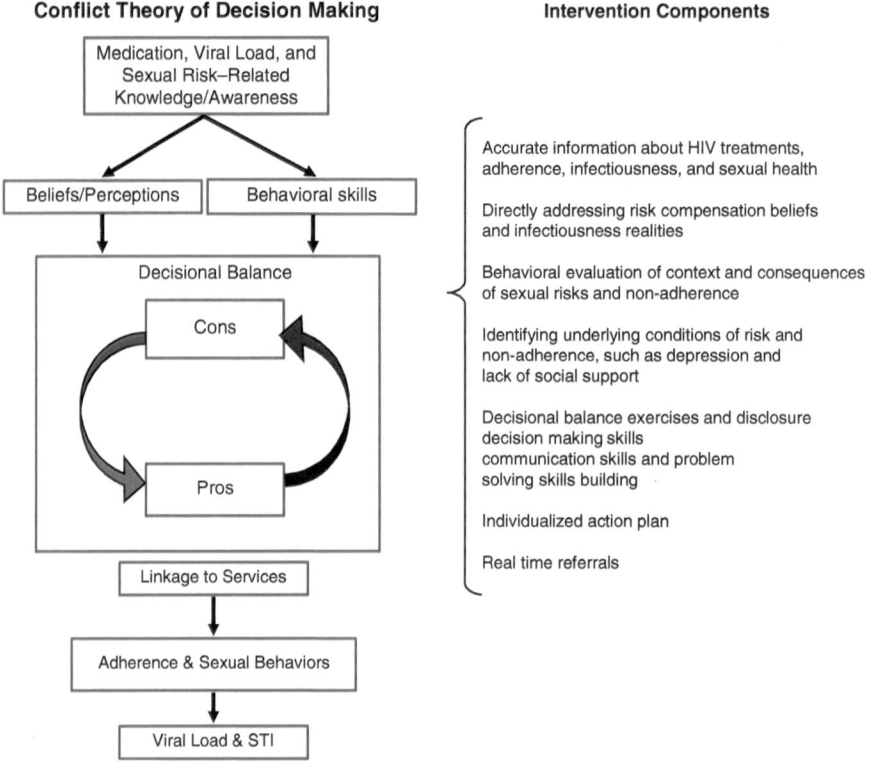

Fig. 3.6 Conflict Theory of Decision Making-based conceptual framework for the In The Mix intervention

behavioral factors that undermine both medication and safer sex adherence, such as mood, substance use, social relations, and environmental factors. We also integrated the groups in terms of gender, with men and women mixed in the same groups regardless of sexual orientation. We also used both individual counseling and small group sessions for the intervention delivery; starting with a one-on-one counseling session, followed by five group sessions, and ending with an individual counseling session. The intervention manual for In The Mix is included in Chap. 4.

In The Mix was based on Conflict Theory of Decision Making. As shown in Fig. 3.6, this model directly addresses beliefs and perceptions in an effort to impact perceived pros and cons of conflicting decisions. The intervention components are keyed to each level of decision-making to ultimately improve treatment and risk behavior outcomes. Guided by this model, the initial individual counseling session worked to set personal treatment and prevention goals for the upcoming group. This session was held by one of the two group facilitators and was aimed to motivate the participant to attend the groups, answer their questions, and address any concerns about the groups. After participants completed their individual session, they attended the first group session, which focused on building cohesion and trust. The facilitators explained that both risk reduction and improving health through treatment were the goals of In The Mix. They also explained how these two goals are related—how treatments reduce viral load to improve health and can make people less infectious if they are adherent and free of STI. The session included a team-building game designed to educate participants about the basics of HIV transmission, treatment resistance, and viral load. Myths and facts about infectiousness were covered in detail. The second group session focused on understanding HIV treatment including deciding when to start medications. Decisional balance exercises were applied to treatment decisions and sexual relationships in contexts of detectable and undetectable viral loads. Group session 3 focused entirely on sexual decision-making under various nuanced conditions of moods, substance use, relationships, HIV status disclosure, treatment status, and viral load. Group 4 aimed to build treatment and safer sex decision skills in relation to substance use. A core activity had participants wear vision-disorienting, or "drunken," goggles to simulate intoxication while filling a pillbox with mints and then applying a condom to a penis model. Participants were then trained in medication management and safer sex strategies including male and female condoms. Group 5 emphasized treatment adherence to reduce viral load and strategies to increase STI detection and treatment. The final individual counseling session occurred within 1 week of the last group. This session also developed a personalized plan for treatment decisions, adherence, and safer sex.

The trial randomly assigned 436 people living with HIV to either the In The Mix group or a time and contact matched health-behavior comparison intervention. Participants were followed for 9 months with over 90% retention. Medication adherence was monitored with monthly unannounced home-based pill counts and sexual behavior was assessed in computerized interviews. In addition, viral load and STI were assessed by self-report during the computerized interviews. The intervention outcomes from In The Mix were encouraging [173]. Results showed that the In The Mix groups demonstrated significantly better medication adherence over the course of the follow-up. Adherence for the comparison group remained around 70% of pills taken, while the In The Mix group increased from below 70 to over 80% adherence. These differences were sustained over the follow-up (see Fig. 3.7). Similar results were observed for sexual risk behavior changes as well as targeted adherence strategies, safer sex strategies, and infectiousness beliefs. Although groups did not differ in their reported changes in viral load, analyses for acquiring a new bacterial STI aggregated over the 9 months post-intervention showed a significant difference between conditions; fewer participants in the integrated intervention (5/143 sexually active, 3.5%) reported new STI than the comparison intervention (13/150 sexually active, 8.6%). Although the STI outcome was limited by a self-report measure, it demonstrates that integrated behavioral interventions have the potential to achieve the two primary outcomes necessary for TasP to succeed— antiretroviral adherence and controlling sexually transmitted coinfections.

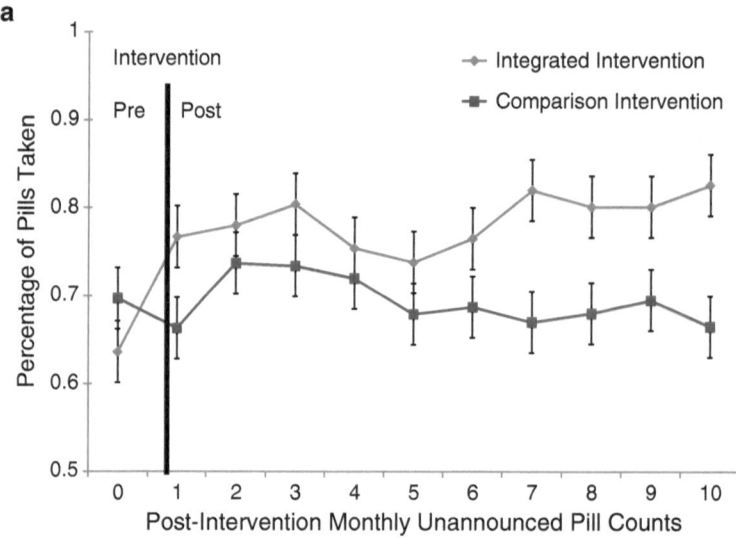

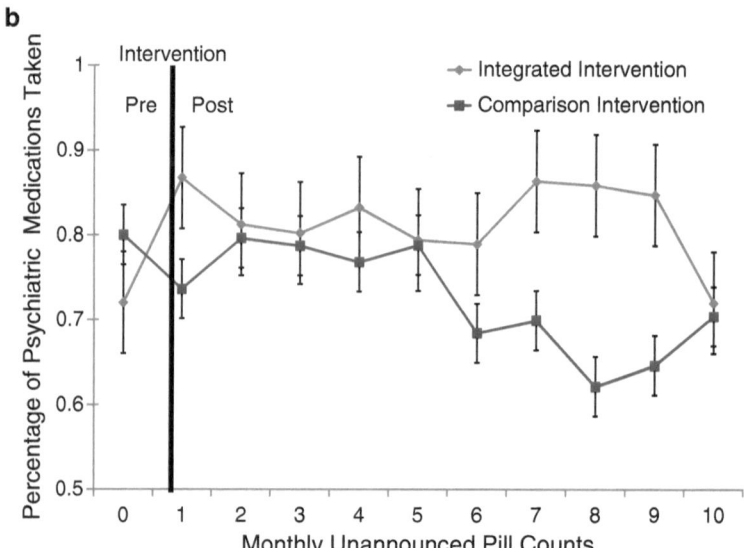

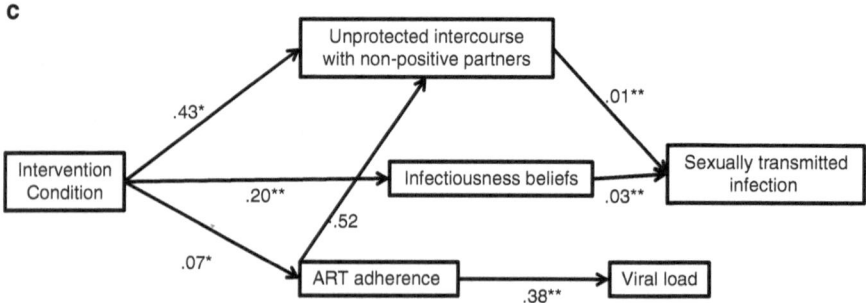

**Fig. 3.7** (**a**) Unannounced pill count HIV treatment pill count and (**b**) psychiatric medication adherence for the In The Mix intervention and control condition and (**c**) structural model of intervention concepts and outcomes (Kalichman et al. [173])

## The Big Picture

The HIV prevention revolution is marked by an influx of tools that can be leveraged against the virus. The task at hand is to integrate these new tools with behavioral strategies that optimize their impact. Figure 3.8 illustrates just one of many paths for the future of HIV prevention. Scaling up a comprehensive HIV prevention program will require outreach to those at greatest risk and mobilizing communities. Energizing communities for HIV prevention at this stage of the epidemic will certainly not be easy. AIDS is no longer seen as a crisis. In fact, AIDS apathy is at an all time high. In addition, the barriers to prevention that we encountered for years are still with us, including stigma, addictions, poverty, apathy, denial, and avoidance. Fortunately, we can draw on 30 years of community interventions to orchestrate an engagement strategy. The National Institute on Drug Abuse Cooperative Agreement and CDC's Community Demonstration Projects, for example, developed outreach, engagement, social marketing, and venue intercept strategies that are as applicable today as they were in the 1990s. These technologies can be tailored for use in targeted community services that intersect with the highest risk populations, including bars, shelters, STI clinics, substance abuse treatment centers, mental health services, and reproductive health clinics. Concentrating resources on risk populations in cities with the highest HIV prevalence will prove most cost-efficient. HIV testing can be delivered at point of contact using existing procedures and technologies. However, a smart approach

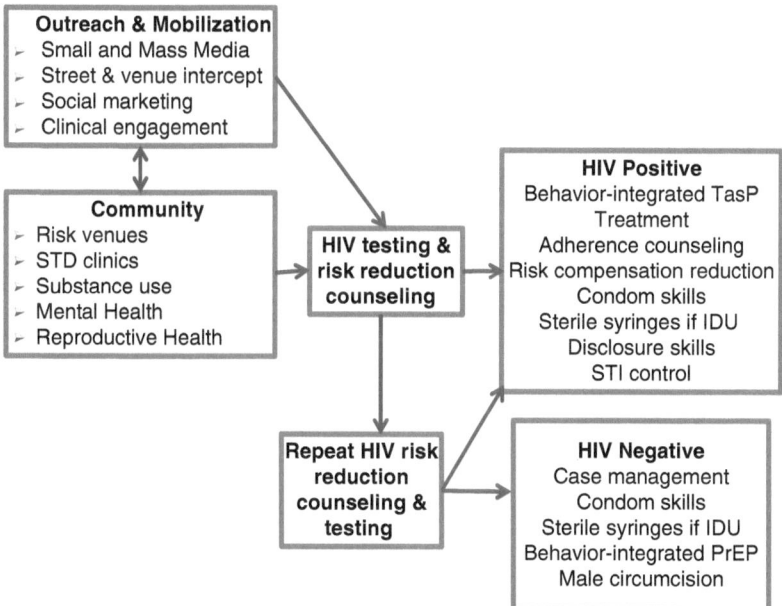

**Fig. 3.8** Comprehensive framework for HIV prevention

to HIV prevention will not miss opportunities to deliver counseling with testing. Brief risk reduction counseling models that capitalize on the teachable moment must be reinvigorated and integrated with testing. In addition, individuals who repeatedly test HIV negative should be engaged in risk assessments to determine the best approach to primary prevention to meet their needs. There are now multiple prevention options for uninfected persons and more choices are coming. The challenge to prevention services is to develop access points for intensive behavioral interventions that include condoms, syringe exchange, PrEP, circumcision, etc.

For those who test HIV positive, TasP should be offered within a broader array of prevention services. This Brief has offered one way forward for developing a behaviorally integrated approach to TasP. There will be obstacles. Some politicians will refuse to pay for treatments for people who are not yet sick. Naysayers will raise concerns about adherence, potential for abuse, irresponsible behavior, and recklessness. To many of us these fights will be reminiscent of abstinence-only sex education, the Federal ban on syringe access, failures to invest in prevention, delinking counseling from testing, and framing circumcision as genital mutilation. We should expect the same flavor of opposition to TasP. We should also expect gravitation toward the easy path of merely dispensing pills as prevention. We must, however, resist these barriers and take a smarter approach to TasP. To avoid repeating mistakes of the past, HIV prevention must pivot away from a single-minded view of prevention technologies and implement TasP within a potent behavioral framework.

# Appendix
# Resources: In The Mix Intervention Manual

## In The Mix

### Decision Condition Session Outline and Guides

### Session 1

## SESSION ONE GOALS

- ➤ Introduction: Goals and expectations of the group
- ➤ Establish group cohesiveness and trust
- ➤ Explore group members who are as individuals living with HIV
- ➤ Establish "community" norms
- ➤ Introduce decision making/decisional balance

## FACILITATOR: Introduction (5 min)

*Welcome to In The Mix. My name is (fill in) and this is (fill in) and we will be your group facilitators for this project. For those of you who have never participated in one of our projects, SHARE Project is a research group that is a part of the University of Connecticut and works with the AIDS Survival Project. We conduct educational research to develop programs that help people with HIV live healthier lives. The SHARE Project has been doing programs focused on HIV/AIDS since 1995. Our programs are usually fun as well as educational. People generally come back and look forward to the next program.*

S.C. Kalichman, *HIV Treatments as Prevention (TasP):*
*Primer for Behavior-Based Implementation*, SpringerBriefs in Public Health,
DOI 10.1007/978-1-4614-5119-8, © Seth C. Kalichman 2013

## ACTIVITY: Group members introduce themselves (5 min)

*Now that you know who we are. I'm going to ask you to introduce yourself to the rest of the group. I'm going to ask you to tell us your name and what prompted you to sign up for this program.*

## ACTIVITY: Group Rules (10 min)

*Coming to a group, with people you do not know and not knowing what to expect, can be uncomfortable. We want everybody in this group to feel comfortable. One way to make sure everyone is comfortable is to make sure that everyone is on the same page. We would like to establish some group rules or ground rules not to dictate what people should and should not do, but to make sure that we are all comfortable coming to the group.*

*Think about what kinds of things that we could include that would make you and others feel comfortable when you come to the group. The first thing we like to start with is confidentiality. Confidentiality means that what is said in here stays in here. What other things can we add to our group rules?*

Have the group members generate other group rules and write them on the newsprint.
     Be sure that the group includes:

- No judgments
- No put downs
- Respect each other
- Right to ask questions
- Right to pass, no drugs or alcohol
- No weapons or violence

*Thank you for participating in this exercise. We have learned each others names, but we would like to get to know more about each other. The way we are going to get to know more about each other is through our first activity.*

## HOUSEKEEPING

*Thank you for being willing to participate in these groups. Your willingness to come to group and share with each other will help us to develop better programs for others who are living with HIV.*

*The In The Mix group will meet five times over the next 3 weeks. We will meet on (day of the week) at (time of day). Each week we will do activities, watch videos, and have discussions about things that can help us live healthier with HIV. This group is closed which means we will not be allowing any other people to join our group. We may lose some people if someone does not decide to come back, but we hope that everyone will return because the groups are a lot of fun as well as educational. We will begin each group promptly at (fill in). Half way through the group we will take a short break.*

Facilitators should provide participants with general information about participating in the group such as:

Where bathrooms are located
What type of snacks will be provided
Where to go if they need to smoke
Cleaning up after the group
How the on-time lottery works
Guidelines for coming late to group or leaving early

## ACTIVITY: WHO AM I CUE CARDS (15 MIN)

*I am going to give each of you a stack of cards. Each card has a statement on it and one card is blank. Choose three cards which help us to know who you are as a person. You can select three preprinted statements or two preprinted statement cards and use the blank card to make your statement about yourself that is not included. After everyone has had a chance to select their cards, we will go around the room and share.*

*Thank you for participating in this activity. As you can see, we share much more in common than being HIV positive.*

*In The Mix is really about making healthy choices. We call it In The Mix because we aren't going to focus on just one choice like many programs do—either medications or staying safe or alcohol and drugs or feelings and moods or meeting people. In The Mix is about choices—all types of choices.*

*Let's begin by talking about the choices we make. In general what we believe has an effect on what choices and decisions we make. For example, if we believe or maybe someone in our family told us that walking under a ladder will bring us bad luck, we are likely to walk around the ladder. This is no different where our health is concerned. Each day people make decisions based on what they and others believe.*

*We are going to do an activity that looks at what other people believe about HIV and living with HIV and how those beliefs can influence our decisions.*

# ACTIVITY: THE BUZZ IN THE COMMUNITY (25 MIN)

*I am going to read some statements and ask you to go and stand under one of the signs you see on the wall: agree or disagree to indicate what you think others in the community believe. Next I am going to ask a few of you to explain why you chose to stand where you are standing.*

Read each statement to the participants. Give the participants time to move to indicate what they think others believe about the statement. Ask a few participants to share...

- How do you know others believe this?
- How does this belief impact you and other people who are HIV positive?

---

**Statements for participants:**

It is possible for a person with an undetectable viral load to transmit the virus to others.

It is easy for people to remember to take their medications.

If an HIV positive man has an undetectable viral load, he is less likely to infect his partner if he is the insertive partner.

An HIV positive woman with an undetectable viral load is less likely to infect her partner.

If an HIV positive person wants to go drinking for the evening they should stop taking their medications for the evening.

If an HIV positive person has risky sex with another HIV positive person, they can become super infected.

---

# DISCUSSION:

Facilitators generate a brief discussion about how others beliefs effects our decision making. **Key point: If a person's belief is faulty or based on inaccurate information, then they are likely to make a decision may affect their health in a negative way.**

# ACTIVITY: FAMILY FEUD GAME (25 MIN)

*We've just seen examples of how what others believe can have an effect on the decisions we make. We often believe that, we are either just like everyone else or we believe we are the only person having this experience. In our research over the past 10 years with people living with HIV in Atlanta, we have collected a lot of information on the experiences of people living with HIV. We are now going to play a game that looks at some of the information. The game is Family Feud—In The Mix Style.*

*Here are the rules: We are going to divide into two teams. You will both be asked a question. Whoever gives the correct answer will go first. You may and should consult with your other team members. Write your answer on the white boards. If you answer the question correctly you will win the point. The next question will be asked of the other team and we will continue until everyone has had a chance to answer a question. At the end of the game we will see who has earned the most points playing Family Feud.*

# FAMILY FEUD QUESTIONS:

What percent of SHARE Project participants say they have stayed in the hospital overnight due to HIV or AIDS? 43%

What percent of SHARE Project participants say they are taking HIV medication? 64%

Which HIV medication is most frequently taken by SHARE Project participants? Combivir 51%

What percent of SHARE Project participants say that they use a pill box to organize their pills? 39%

What percent of SHARE Project participants carry a dose of their medications with them on most days? 52%

For SHARE Project participants who are taking HIV medications, what percent have not missed taking a dose of their medications in the past week? 58%

What percent of SHARE Project participants say they are currently drinking alcohol? 50%

What percent of SHARE Project participants say they have used street drugs during the past 3 months? 25%

What percent of SHARE Project participants say they have had an STD? 63%

What percent of SHARE Project participants say that it is difficult to tell their sex partners that they have HIV? 51%

## DISCUSSION: FAMILY FEUD

Facilitators lead a brief discussion on the information extracted from the game questions. Possible lead-off questions include:

What did you think of some of the information that was presented?
Did any of the information come as a surprise to you?

*We've looked at what the community beliefs are and what the community is doing. In addition to understanding what is happening in our community, it is important to understand what our own beliefs are, because they will often influence the decisions we make in life.*

*Now let's spend some time talking about how we make decisions and how we can make decisions that help us remain healthy and have the most positive health outcome for us. We make many decisions each day, but often times we believe that we do not have any choices in the decisions that we make, when in reality we didn't take time to weigh the choices we had.*

*We like to look at this as a decisional balance or weighing as Pros and Cons. We can weigh the choices of every decision and every choice we make has Pros and Cons. When we take time to examine the Pros and Cons before we make a decision, it can result in a more positive outcome.*

## ACTIVITY: DECISIONAL BALANCE OF COMING TO GROUP (10 MIN)

*I am going to demonstrate how we work through a decisional balance by asking you to come up with all of the pros and cons for coming to this group today. Remember that your reasons may differ from others in the group and that is okay.*

|                      | Pros | Cons |
| -------------------- | ---- | ---- |
| Coming to Group      |      |      |
| Not Coming to group  |      |      |

*As you can see there are many valid reasons for people to make the decision to come to group or not to come to group. By using a decisional balance, we can weigh out the decision and come to a decision that is best for us individually.*

## ACTIVITY: MOVIE CLIP-BOAT TRIP (5 MIN)

*Let's finish up today by watching a video of two people who make decisions based on something they believed themselves or someone else believed.*

# DISCUSSION: PROCESS VIDEO TAPE

## SESSION WRAP UP

- What did you think of the first session?
- Have each participant complete a session questionnaire
- Let each participant know that they will receive their group payment
- The time and date of the next session
- On time lottery

# Session 2

## SESSION TWO GOALS

➢ HIV medication treatment education
➢ How treatment affects decision making regarding partners and relationships
➢ Medication update
➢ Barriers to effective decision making around treatment and relationships

## REVIEW LAST GROUP (5 MIN)

*Welcome back to our second group. Last time we met we learned how our decisions are influenced by others. Then we played Family Feud which demonstrated what others in the community are actually doing versus what we thought they were doing. Finally, we discussed the decisional balance and looked at the pros and cons of making decisions. Today we are going to be looking at decision making around treatment and relationships.*

*In order for us to make good decisions the first thing we need to do is to understand the difference between what information is a myth and what information is fact. Remember in the last group we played Family Feud where we looked at what people in the community were actually doing versus what we thought they were doing. Today we are going to talk about medications and what we think are the facts about medications and what the facts actually are.*

# ACTIVITY MYTH AND FACTS GAME (20 MIN)

Facilitator explains that he/she is going to read a statement from a card and participants will decide whether the statement is a myth or fact. Once a statement is read, participants discuss whether they believe it is a fact of myth. After discussion facilitator will give the factual information on the inside of the card if it hasn't been given by the participants. Each card should be thoroughly discussed.

**Myths and Facts:**
If I am taking medications for HIV and I am going to go out drinking, it is better for me to stop taking my medications for that day.
**FACT**: It is very rare for alcohol to adversely interact with HIV medications. It is better to never miss a dose of HIV medications even if you drink alcohol.

Being undetectable means that I don't have to be as careful about infecting my partners.
**FACT**: Having an undetectable viral load sometimes means that your genital fluids (semen or vaginal fluids) are also undetectable…but not always. Even when your genital fluids are undetectable, HIV can still be transmitted by the small amounts that are there and the HIV that has infected your cells in those fluids.

If I miss a dose of my HIV medication I should take a double dose the next time.
**FACT**: In almost all cases, HIV medications should not be double dosed. If you miss a dose, take it late and take the next dose when it is time. If it is close to the time for the next dose, just take that dose.

All HIV treatments work in the same way to stop the virus.
**FACT**: Each class of antiretroviral medications works on a different part of the HIV reproduction cycle. That is why combinations of drugs are so effective—they hit HIV in different ways.

It is a good idea to stop taking all medications now and then to clean your body.
**FACT**: Interrupting treatment without the supervision of your doctor, such as drug holidays, can be a serious risk for developing treatment resistance and should be avoided.

A person who has an undetectable viral load no longer has AIDS.
**FACT**: A person who has AIDS has a T-cell CD4 cell count under 200 cells or has been diagnosed with an AIDS-related opportunistic disease regardless of their viral load. Having undetectable viral load does not change an AIDS diagnosis but can help slow the disease process.

When the viral load is undetectable in the blood, it is also undetectable in the semen and the vaginal fluids.
**FACT**: Viral load in blood and genital fluids are often related; when one is undetectable so too is the other. But not always, and when a person has an STD or other cause of infection in their genitals the viral load in their semen or vaginal fluids can be very high even when they are undetectable in their blood.

T-cells and CD4 cells are two different things.

**FACT**: No, T-Cells and CD4 cells are two different names for the same immune cells.

In Georgia, as long as you use a condom, you do not have to tell a person you are HIV positive.

**FACT**: HIV-infected people are legally required to disclose their infection status to another person prior to engaging in sexual activity or sharing injection drug needles with that person. (O.C.G.A. 16-5-60)

If you are HIV positive it is safe to have unprotected sex with another HIV positive person.

**FACT**: There may be risks for a person with HIV getting a different strain of HIV. Combining HIV types may cause superinfection—more virulent strains of the virus. Most risk comes from the potential for other STDs, or coinfection, that can cause serious health problems in people with HIV.

There is no such thing as HIV drug resistance.

**FACT**: HIV can rapidly develop resistance to antiretroviral medications. Once resistant, HIV is no longer suppressed by that drug. The development of resistant viral strains is one of the main reasons for failure of antiretroviral therapy. If there is resistance to several drug classes, the number of alternative treatment regimens is limited and the virological success of subsequent therapies, or so-called salvage regimens, may be only short-lived.

Using the withdrawal method will protect my partner if we don't use condoms.

**FACT**: Withdrawal (or pulling out before ejaculation) may limit the amount of semen a partner is exposed to. But there is HIV in precum fluids and sometimes men will ejaculate before pulling out. So there may be only limited protection offered by withdrawal.

## ACTIVITY: ARV VIDEO-HIV RESISTANCE (15 MIN)

*We now know more of the facts about HIV, resistance, and transmission. Let's learn some of the facts about the medications to treat HIV. It is important to understand how they work before you decide to take HIV medication or not. Let's watch a film about your immune system and antiretroviral therapy.*

Facilitator shows video on how ARV's work to support the immune system and suppress the virus.

- CD4 cells and how the virus affects the CD4 cells
- Viral load and how it is affected by medication
- How the medications attack the virus at different stages

Following the video, facilitators generate a discussion about the information covered in the video. Possible lead-off questions include:

What did you think of some of the information that was presented?
Did any of the information come as a surprise to you?

*The Journal of Test Positive Aware Network publishes a HIV Drug Guide each year. It is an excellent resource for you to have. It provides information on the latest drugs used to treat HIV, including dosing information, side effects, and information on potential drug interaction. Remember we said that in order to make better decisions, you need to have the facts. This Journal will give you some of those facts which will help you to make your decision about going on or off of medication.*

Facilitator passes out a copy of TPAN special edition on medications.

*Understanding how the medications for HIV work is not enough to make a decision whether to take them or not. There are many other things to consider, such as side effects.*

## ACTIVITY: HANDS ON VIRUS (10 MIN)

*To illustrate the strength of HIV medications and how they work to suppress HIV let's do a brief activity. I would like each of you to choose one of these cards—Non-nucleoside, Nucleoside, Protease Inhibitor, or Entry Inhibitor. I am going to sit in a chair in the center of the room and I am going to be HIV. I want all of you who have an Entry Inhibitor card to place one hand on my shoulder. As I try to stand up, I want each of you to work on holding me down with one hand. Now I would like the Nucleosides to put one of your hands on my shoulder along with the Entry Inhibitors and try to hold me down as I stand up. Let's do this again with all who are the Non-nucleosides. Using one hand all of you try to hold me down as I stand up. Finally I want the Protease Inhibitors to join in and try to suppress me, using one hand. As more of you are added, you are more effective at holding me down or suppressing me.*

*Now let's become non-adherent to ARVs. We are going to reverse this exercise with the Protease Inhibitors removing your hands first. Now Non-nucleosides, Nucleosides, and finally Entry Inhibitors remove your hands.*

## DISCUSSION

- Point out the benefit of combination drug therapies
- Importance of following your prescribed regimen
- Discuss the most popular drug combinations (according to SHARE Project data) for people living in Atlanta

# ACTIVITY: HIV MEDICATION DECISIONAL BALANCE (10 MIN)

*Let's work through a decisional balance about whether to take medication or not. Remember there may be many different Pros and Cons for taking medication or for not taking medication.*

# DISCUSSION: UNDETECTABLE VIRAL LOAD (5 MIN)

Following the Hands on Virus activity, facilitators lead a short discussion on having an undetectable viral load and what it really means. Facilitators can use the myth/fact cards that contain the undetectable viral load statements to begin the discussion.

*After being on ARV therapy, some people may find that their viral load is undetectable. When your viral load is determined to be undetectable, this means that there are not enough copies of the virus in your blood to be detected at the time of the blood test.*

*How does having an undetectable viral load affect someone in terms of the decisions that they make?*

○ **Clarify that viral load refers to the level of virus found in the blood**
○ **Explain that current test can only measure down to a certain degree**
○ **Explain it is believed that a person is less infectious when undetectable**
○ **Explain that viral load can be influenced by infection of a STD**

# SCENARIO ACTIVITY (30 MIN)

*Let's read two different scenarios. For each scenario I want you to think about the sexual decisional balance faced by the lead character. Then we will work through a decisional balance for the scenario.*

> **Marta's Scenario**
> Marta has been HIV+ for 12 years and has been on meds for the past 3 years. At her last doctor visit she was told that her viral load was undetectable. Marta was so happy that she decided to celebrate by going out. While at a bar she ran into Joe who she's been attracted to for many years. She believes Joe may be HIV+, but she does not know. Joe does not know Marta's HIV status. They hit it off and decide to go back to her place. Joe puts the moves on Marta and lets her know that he wants to have sex with her.

# MARTA'S DECISIONAL BALANCE (HAVE SEX/NOT HAVE SEX)

*Facilitator works through the decisional balance for*
*Marta and Joe to have sex on newsprint.*

# DISCUSSION POINTS:

How does Mary's undetectable status affect her decision to disclose or not to disclose? (include discussion of Georgia Law)

How does her undetectable status effect her decision to have protected or unprotected sex?

How does her undetectable status affect the likely hood of her infecting her partner if they have unprotected sex?

How does her undetectable status effect her decision to select Joe as a HIV-negative partner?

# HARRY'S DECISIONAL BALANCE (HAVE SAFE SEX/NOT HAVE SAFE SEX)

*Facilitator works through the decisional*
*balance for Harry and Dick to have safe sex on newsprint.*

**Harry's Scenario**
Harry has been HIV+ for 4 years, has an undetectable viral load and was recently laid off from his job. This has been very difficult for him because he loved his job. While in the grocery store shopping for comfort food, he ran into his old lover, Dick, who he never quite got over. Dick is also HIV+ and they both know each other's statuses. Harry and Dick decide to go to Starbucks to catch up. After a latte and great conversation, Dick invites Harry to his place for dinner in the hopes that they can rekindle their sexual relationship.

# DISCUSSION POINTS

How does Harry's viral load affect his decision to sex?
How does Harry's viral load affect his likelihood that he will reinfect Dick?
Should Harry consider being top or bottom with Dick?

# MAPS (10 MIN)

*We have talked about how what we believe, what others believe, and having an undetectable viral load can affect our decision making. Now we are going to explore another aspect of decision making. It is what we call MAPS. MAPS stands for Moods, Alcohol and other substances, People, and Situations. When we are on a trip, we often use road maps to help us get to our final destination. But it is not enough to have a map, it's really up to the driver to get you where you are going. The MAPS that we are going to talk to you about influence our decision making. By understanding our own MAPS, we will be better decision makers.*

# ACTIVITY: LIST MAPS

*Every decision we make is influenced by our Mood, Alcohol or other substances we may be using, People around us and the Situation we are in. Let's begin by coming up with a list for each part of the MAPS—Mood, Alcohol and other substances, People, and Situations that affect our decision making. Remember that everyone may have different components to their own MAPS that affect their decision making.*

*Now look at the list and identify which one of these things is the driver in your decision making or has the most influence in your decision making. This influence can be either positive or negative.*

*If we understand our own personal MAPS it will help us to make decisions that have more positive outcomes.*

# UNTIL WE MEET AGAIN

*Before you come back to group next time I would like you to be aware of the decisions that you make and think about the MAPS in your life and how your MAPS influenced your decisions.*

## SESSION WRAP UP:

- What did you think of the second session? Do you have any questions before we conclude?
- Session questionnaire
- Let each participant know that they will receive their group payment
- The time and date of the next session
- On time lottery

# Session 3

## Session 3 Goals

➢ Participants will learn to identify different components of MAPS
➢ Participants will learn how to identify the driver for sexual risk and medication decisions

*Last time we met we discussed decision making and how our MAPS or Moods and Feelings, Alcohol and other substances, People, and Situations influence our decision making. We all have MAPS to deal with and just knowing what they are doesn't make them go away. We have to learn strategies to help manage them. We must first however, determine which of the MAPS has the greatest influence or who is the driver. We are now going to watch a movie clip that will help you practice identifying the different components of MAPS and finding strategies to manage them. The first clip involves a People influence around a medication decision.*

*Let's take a look at an interaction between a patient and his doctor. Roy comes to see his doctor because he is not feeling well. His doctor diagnoses him with advanced HIV. Roy does not know much about HIV or what to do.*

## Activity: Dr. Smith and Roy Video Clip (People Influence—Medication)

After viewing the video clip, facilitator leads the participants in a discussion to MAPS the situation. Possible discussion questions:

- Do you think this doctor was helpful in assisting this patient with the decision to take medication or not?
- Was this doctor easy to talk with?
- What about this patient–doctor interaction influenced the patient's decision to adhere to their medication or to not adhere to their medication?
- What if that patient is already taking medication but the patient is not adhering to their medication regimen?

## Strategies Brainstorm

- Have any of you experienced any of these situations
- What strategies they used to solve the problem. Remind participants about the decisional balance for taking and not taking ARV's that was done earlier.

**List the strategies that participants used to solve these problems. Facilitators should go around the room and ask each participant to select a strategy from the list, they would use if they were to find themselves in a similar situation in the future. Facilitators use role-plays, etc. to help other participants practice using these strategies for themselves.**

## Activity: Dr. Smith and Roy (2 min)

Facilitators lead a discussion around the video clip for other influences on the scenario (what if it were a different driver or the driver changed). Participants should brainstorm strategies for dealing with these influences.

- ➢ Drug and alcohol problem
- ➢ Multiple sex partners
- ➢ History of depression
- ➢ What else might make a difference?

## Activity: Pat's MAPS Scenario Cards (20 min)

*You will each be given a set of MAPS cards. I am going to read a scenario. I would like you to think about which component of the MAPS had the greatest influence or driving force on the person making the decision. Then I want you to hold up the card to indicate what you think.*

## Pat's Scenario

Pat's mom recently died after a long illness in which Pat was the primary caregiver. Pat has been really struggling with this loss because their relationship was more than parent and child, they were best friends. Two days after the funeral Pat went out to a bar to have a drink and hopefully feel better. While there Pat runs into Jessie, an old lover that Pat has always had feelings for. Jessie and Pat continue drinking and having a good time talking about all of the wonderful things they did in the past. They eventually go back to Jessie's house. It was in Jessie's place where they both believe they had their best sex ever. As the night goes on things heat up and Jessie and Pat have sex again.

## Discussion

Process with participants their different choices and why they made those choices.

- MAPS have influence on our decision making
- Each person has to decide for him /her self which of the MAPS is driving
- Identify the MAPS for Pat's scenario

  - Mood—sadness and grieving
  - Alcohol—alcohol
  - Person—old lover, Jessie
  - Situation—familiar sex spot
  - Ask each group member to identify what is the driver for Pat.

- After each group member shares what they think the driver is for that situation, remind group members that

  - For each person the driver can be different
  - It is important to figure out what your driver is in any given situation
  - There is always a driver in any situation even though all of these things play a part

## Activity: DeAndre and Martin Video (People Influence—Sex) (30 min)

*Now let's take a look at another scene that involves a People influence for a sexual relationship decision. In this next scene DeAndre and Martin are attracted to each other, but both have other people they are involved with. DeAndre is HIV positive and he believes Martin is negative but doesn't know his status. DeAndre has not told Martin his HIV status. They are at a party with women they are involved with.*

## Strategies Brainstorm

- Have any of you experienced a situation like this or can you imagine being in a situation like this?
- What strategies have they used or could this person have used to solve the problem.

**List the strategies that participants used to solve these problems. Facilitators should go around the room and ask each participant to select a strategy from the list, they would use if they were to find themselves in a similar situation in the future. Facilitators use role-plays, etc. to help other participants practice using these strategies for themselves.**

## Activity: Deandre and Martin Video (2 min)

*Now let's think about the scene we just watched. Facilitators lead a discussion around the video clip for other influences on the scenario (what if it were a different driver or the driver changed). What if...*

> ➢ *Martin is also HIV positive and has not told Deandre*
> ➢ *Deandre has an undetectable viral load*
> ➢ *They had not been drinking*
> ➢ *What else might make a difference?*

## Activity: The Married Man (Situation Influence) (30 min)

*Now lets watch a video that involves a Situation Influence. In this scene an HIV positive married man who found out today that he has an undetectable viral load is attracted to a woman whose status he does not know. He has not disclosed his HIV status to her but he knows he wants to be with her. He meets her for dinner and to talk.*

## Strategies Brainstorm

- Have any of you experienced a situation like this or can you imagine being in a situation like this?
- What strategies have they used or could this person have used to solve the problem.

**List the strategies that participants used to solve these problems. Facilitators should go around the room and ask each participant to select a strategy from the list, they would use if they were to find themselves in a similar situation in the future. Facilitators use role-plays, etc. to help other participants practice using these strategies for themselves.**

## Activity: The Married Man (2 min)

*Now lets think about the scene we just watched. Facilitators lead a discussion around the video clip for other influences on the scenario (what if it were a different driver or the driver changed). What if...*

> ➢ *It was time for him to take his medication*
> ➢ *His viral load was not undetectable*

> *She was drinking alcohol instead of coffee*
> *What else might make a difference?*

## Session Wrap Up:

- What did you think of the third session? Do you have any questions before we conclude?
- Let each participant know that they will receive their group payment
- Complete session questionnaire
- The time and date of the next session
- On time lottery

# Session 4

## Session Goals

> Education and behavioral skills training on the relationship between substance use and risk behavior
> Education and behavioral skills training on the relationship between substance use and adherence to medication
> Education and behavioral skills training on the relationship between mood/affect and risk behavior
> Education and behavioral skills training on the relationship between mood/affect and adherence to medication

*The last time we were here we identified People and Situation drivers and discussed how they can influence our decisions to take medications and engage in risky sexual relationships. We also brainstormed strategies to manage these influences. Today we are going to identify Mood/Feeling and Alcohol/Substance drivers that can affect medication and sexual relationship decisions. We are going to begin today by watching a video which talks about how drugs and alcohol impact people living with HIV, sexual risk decisions, and decisions to take medication.*

## Activity: Biggest Mess Video (25 min)

## Discussion

- Did you learn anything new about these drugs or their effects on people living with HIV?
- Facilitator reviews effects of drugs using posters.

## Activity: Decisional Balance of Alcohol and Other Substance Use (10 min)

*We now have more information about alcohol and drugs and their effect on people living with HIV. So let's work through a decisional balance on whether to use or not to use.*

Facilitators solicit pros and cons around using alcohol and other substances. Emphasize how using or not using substances can affect your decision making around both sexual behavior and medication adherence.

|  | Pros | Con |
|---|---|---|
| Substance use | Makes you more relaxed, takes away worry, can make you horny, can make you feel less depressed at the time, can | Forget to take medication, interactions with medication, take wrong dose of medication, forget to be safe, cant use condom correctly, impairs decision making |
| No substance use | Makes you more focused, clear judgment, more energy, less depressed | Can be socially isolating, can remain inhibited |

## Activity: Brainstorm Strategies Activity (10 min)

*For some of you, you have already made the decision not to use alcohol or other substances. What are some of the strategies that you have used to help manage alcohol and drug use so that it has a positive outcome on decision making.*

**List the strategies that participants used to solve these problems. Facilitators should go arou nd the room and ask each participant to select a strategy from the list, they would use if they were to find themselves in a similar situation in the future. Facilitators use role-plays, etc. to help other participants practice using these strategies for themselves.**

Be sure to include:

Enter NA program
Enter AA program
Change drug of choice to one that is manageable
Talk with friend or family about drug and alcohol use
Cut down on usage
Enter into a treatment program

## Activity: Impaired Glasses (15 min)

*We are going to split up into pairs. Each pair will be given a pair of glasses that will simulate what it is like to be under the influence of alcohol or other substances. One person will try to put a condom on a penis model and the other person will try to sort Tic Tacs into a pill box while wearing the glasses. The person not wearing the glasses will observe his partner trying to complete the task but is not allowed to help his/her partner. After you have each had the opportunity to complete your task we will come back together as a group and discuss your experiences.*

## Medication Regimen:

**Medication 1—2 pills × three times per day**
**Medication 2—1 pill × two times per day**
**Medication 3—1 pill × one time per day**

## Mood and Feelings Influence

## Activity: Family Feud game (25 min)

*Remember we played the Family Feud game earlier. Now we are going to play Family Feud again. Rather than using data about what previous SHARE Project participants have done, we are going to look at the moods and feelings of previous SHARE Project participants.*

What percentage of the SHARE Project participants said that they felt depressed in the past week? 51%

What percentage of the SHARE Project participants said that they felt lonely in the past week? 49%

What percentage of the SHARE Project participants said that they felt happy in the past week? 69%

What percentage of the SHARE Project participants said that they felt fearful in the past week? 39%

What percentage of the SHARE Project participants said that they enjoyed life in the past week? 63%

What percentage of the SHARE Project participants said that they had a poor appetite in the past week? 30%

What percentage of the SHARE Project participants said that they felt they could not get going in the past week? 40%

What percentage of the SHARE Project participants said that they felt hopeful about the future in the past week?86%

What percentage of the SHARE Project participants said that they felt they had more good times ahead of then than bad times? 80%

What percentage of the SHARE Project participants said that they felt sick there was someone who could help them get to the doctor? 46%

*Feelings and moods can affect medication adherence and sexual risk decisions. The effect can be either positive or negative. Take feeling happy, for example. If you feel happy, you may be more likely to want to stay healthy and you are more likely to take your medication. But if you feel happy you may also want to go and party and be with other people so you may be more likely to take a medication holiday so you can drink and party. Feeling happy with your sexual risk behavior, you may decide to only have sex with condoms because you want to protect your health, but you may also decide to have sex without condoms because you are feeling so happy and carefree that nothing in the world can harm you.*

## Activity: Brainstorm Moods and Strategies (15 min)

*I would like you to come up with a list of moods and feelings that can influence decision making. Then let's decide if these Moods/Feelings influence decisions for medication adherence or sexual risk decisions.*

*Now let's look at some strategies to manage Moods and Feelings that negatively influence our decision making*

**List the strategies that participants used to solve these problems. Facilitators should go around the room and ask each participant to select a strategy from the list, they would use if they were to find themselves in a similar situation in the future. Facilitators use role-plays, etc. to help other participants practice using these strategies for themselves.**

*One strategy for managing your moods and feeling is dealing with the stress in your life and learning how to relax. When a person feels stressed, it affects them not only emotionally, but physically as well. Stress can not only cause you to have headaches and aches in other parts of your body but can also take a real toll on your immune system.*

*In order to learn to relax, you do not need any expensive equipment or special training. Stress reduction can be very short and very inexpensive. Let's watch this clip of someone doing a relaxation exercise while at work.*

## Activity: Video Bad Boys Clip (3 min)

## Activity: Relaxation Exercise (7 min)

Facilitators lead participants through a guided imagery exercise.
Session Wrap Up:

- What did you think of the fourth session? Do you have any questions before we conclude?
- Session questionnaire
- Let each participant know that they will receive their group payment
- The time and date of the next session
- On time lottery

# Session 5

## Session 5 Goals

- ➤ STD education
- ➤ Condom skills education
- ➤ Shopping exercise-strategies for decision making

## Activity: My MAPS

*Over the past few weeks we have talked about how Moods and Feelings, Alcohol and other substances, People, and Situations impact our decision making. Let's put it all together by having each person think about the MAPS that most often get you in trouble. Think about the last time you made a decision and which of the MAPS greatly influenced that decision. It can be any decision, but it would be helpful if it were a sexual or medication decision.*

*Let's go around and share. I would like you to tell us which of the MAPS is the greatest challenge for you. Now, I'd like you to view all the strategies we've generated in this group and determine if there is a strategy listed that would help you manage your MAPS in the future. If you are not pleased with the MAPS that influenced your decision or don't see a strategy that would work for you, let's think of strategies to help you manage those in the future.*

## Activity: STD Puppet Video

*In the first session we discussed the need to have all of the facts or information when making a decision. Now let's look at some of the facts about STD's because STD's can negatively impact people living with HIV.*

## Discussion:

*There are very specific issues for people who are HIV positive and who also have a STD. First all STD's are more difficult to treat when a person's immune system is compromised. Secondly, viral STDs can accelerate or speed up the replication of HIV. Thirdly, ulcer causing STDs make it easier to transmit HIV. Fourthly, Some AIDS conditions result from STDs such as KS and CMV.*

*But one more fact that is very important for people who are trying to make decisions around safer sex for themselves and their partners is that people who are HIV positive and who have a STD are much more infectious EVEN IF YOUR VIRAL LOAD IS LOW.*

## Activity: Love Don't Cost A Thing Video

*We all know that condoms will make sex safer for you and your partner. Let's watch this video of a dad demonstrating how to use condoms to his son.*

## Activity: Decisional Balance for Condom Use

*Let's work through a decisional balance for using and not using condoms.*

## Activity: Participant Condom Demonstration

*We have all been shown how to use condoms before. Today I want you to come up with a creative way to teach condom skills to others. Remember that each demonstration has to hit the key point of correct condom use, such as the reservoir tip. Presentations should be no longer than 5–10 min and may not include use of the mouth or putting the condom on orally.*

Participants are split into two groups and told that they need to come up with a creative way to teach condom skills to the other group. Presentations may not include an oral demonstration. We will have 5–10 min for each presentation. Facilitator should do corrective feedback and make sure that the participants know to use water-based lubricants, etc.

## ACTIVITY: Shopping

*Over the past 5 weeks we have talked a lot about our how moods, alcohol, people, and situations affect our decision making. We have also explored how to better make decisions about whether we want to engage in or continue a certain behavior by using the Decisional Balance. Let's now talk about strategies that will help you maintain your health by taking your medications as prescribed by your physician and that will help you maintain your health when sexually active.*

*Up here you will see different tools or strategies that other people have used to stay healthy. I would like each of you to come and look at what is here and choose what items you think you would use and then afterwards we will go around and discuss how you will use each of those items. Yes you get to keep what you choose, but you must be able to state why you chose it, identify strategies to use it effectively and how you will mix it into your day.*

Pill boxes
Condoms
STD brochures
Watches with alarm
Condom key chains
Pillbox key chains
Medication Pocket Planner
Post it notes
Bracelets

Participants fill out their form for what they want. Each person has to process with the group

What they chose
How it will impacted by MAPS

**Group Ending**

# References

1. Kalichman SC, Belcher L, Cherry C, Williams E. Primary prevention of sexually transmitted HIV infections: transferring behavioral research to community programs. J Prim Prev. 1997;18:149–72.
2. Hanenberg RS, Rojanapithayakorn W, Kunasol P, Sokal DC. Impact of Thailand's HIV-control programme as indicated by the decline of sexually transmitted diseases. Lancet. 1994;344(8917):243–5. Epub 23 July 1994.
3. Stoneburner RL, Low-Beer D. Sexual partner reductions explain human immunodeficiency virus declines in Uganda: comparative analyses of HIV and behavioural data in Uganda, Kenya, Malawi, and Zambia. Int J Epidemiol. 2004;33(3):624. Epub 12 June 2004.
4. Slutkin G, Okware S, Naamara W, Sutherland D, Flanagan D, Carael M, et al. How Uganda reversed its HIV epidemic. AIDS Behav. 2006;10(4):351–60. Epub 22 July 2006.
5. Merson M. Uganda's HIV/AIDS Epidemic: Guest Editorial. AIDS Behav. 2006;10:333–4.
6. Skoler-Karpoff S, Ramjee G, Ahmed K, Altini L, Plagianos MG, Friedland B, et al. Efficacy of Carraguard for prevention of HIV infection in women in South Africa: a randomised, double-blind, placebo-controlled trial. Lancet. 2008;372(9654):1977–87. Epub 9 Nov 2008.
7. Dunne EF, Whitehead S, Sternberg M, Thepamnuay S, Leelawiwat W, McNicholl JM, et al. Suppressive acyclovir therapy reduces HIV cervicovaginal shedding in HIV- and HSV-2-infected women, Chiang Rai, Thailand. J Acquir Immune Defic Syndr. 2008;49(1):77–83. Epub 1 Aug 2008.
8. Celum C, Wald A, Hughes J, Sanchez J, Reid S, Delany-Moretlwe S, et al. Effect of aciclovir on HIV-1 acquisition in herpes simplex virus 2 seropositive women and men who have sex with men: a randomised, double-blind, placebo-controlled trial. Lancet. 2008;371(9630):2109–19. Epub 24 June 2008.
9. Watson-Jones D, Weiss HA, Rusizoka M, Changalucha J, Baisley K, Mugeye K, et al. Effect of herpes simplex suppression on incidence of HIV among women in Tanzania. N Engl J Med. 2008;358(15):1560–71. Epub 14 Mar 2008.
10. El-Bassel N, Jemmott JB, Landis JR, Pequegnat W, Wingood GM, Wyatt GE, et al. National Institute of Mental Health Multisite Eban HIV/STD Prevention Intervention for African American HIV Serodiscordant Couples: a cluster randomized trial. Arch Intern Med. 2010;170(17):1594–601. Epub 14 July 2010.
11. Hallett TB, Singh K, Smith JA, White RG, Abu-Raddad LJ, Garnett GP. Understanding the impact of male circumcision interventions on the spread of HIV in southern Africa. PLoS One. 2008;3(5):e2212. Epub 22 May 2008.
12. Williams BG, Lloyd-Smith JO, Gouws E, Hankins C, Getz WM, Hargrove J, et al. The potential impact of male circumcision on HIV in Sub-Saharan Africa. PLoS Med. 2006;3(7):e262. Epub 11 July 2006.

13. Noar SM. Behavioral interventions to reduce HIV-related sexual risk behavior: review and synthesis of meta-analytic evidence. AIDS Behav. 2008;12(3):335–53. Epub 27 Sept 2007.

14. Scott-Sheldon LA, Huedo-Medina TB, Warren MR, Johnson BT, Carey MP. Efficacy of behavioral interventions to increase condom use and reduce sexually transmitted infections: a meta-analysis, 1991 to 2010. J Acquir Immune Defic Syndr. 2011;58(5):489–98. Epub 16 Nov 2011.

15. Scott-Sheldon LA, Fielder RL, Carey MP. Sexual risk reduction interventions for patients attending sexually transmitted disease clinics in the United States: a meta-analytic review, 1986 to early 2009. Ann Behav Med. 2010;40(2):191–204. Epub 24 July 2010.

16. Lagakos SW, Gable AR. Challenges to HIV prevention–seeking effective measures in the absence of a vaccine. N Engl J Med. 2008;358(15):1543–5. Epub 12 Apr 2008.

17. Padian NS, McCoy SI, Balkus JE, Wasserheit JN. Weighing the gold in the gold standard: challenges in HIV prevention research. AIDS. 2010;24(5):621–35 Epub 25 Feb 2010.

18. Padian NS, van der Straten A, Ramjee G, Chipato T, de Bruyn G, Blanchard K, et al. Diaphragm and lubricant gel for prevention of HIV acquisition in southern African women: a randomised controlled trial. Lancet. 2007;370(9583):251–61. Epub 17 July 2007.

19. Koblin B, Chesney M, Coates T. Effects of a behavioural intervention to reduce acquisition of HIV infection among men who have sex with men: the EXPLORE randomised controlled study. Lancet. 2004;364(9428):41–50. Epub 6 July 2004.

20. Chesney MA, Koblin BA, Barresi PJ, Husnik MJ, Celum CL, Colfax G, et al. An individually tailored intervention for HIV prevention: baseline data from the EXPLORE Study. Am J Public Health. 2003;93(6):933–8. Epub 30 May 2003.

21. Kamb M, Fishbein M, Douglas J, Rhodes F, Rogers J, Bolan G, et al. Efficacy of risk-reduction counseling to prevent Human Immunodeficiency Virus and Sexually Transmitted Diseases. J Am Med Assoc. 1998;280(13):1161–7.

22. Chesney, M, Coates, T, Koblin, B. A randomized clinical trial of the efficacy of a behavioral intervention to prevent acquisition of HIV among men who have sex with men: HIVNET Protocol No. 015. Available from http://www.hptn.org/research_studies/HIVNET015Study Documents.htm.

23. Stall R, Duran L, Wisniewski SR, Friedman MS, Marshal MP, McFarland W, et al. Running in place: implications of HIV incidence estimates among urban men who have sex with men in the United States and other industrialized countries. AIDS Behav. 2009;13(4):615–29. Epub 12 Feb 2009.

24. Amico KR, Harman JJ, Johnson BT. Efficacy of antiretroviral therapy adherence interventions: a research synthesis of trials, 1996 to 2004. J Acquir Immune Defic Syndr. 2006; 41(3):285–97. Epub 17 Mar 2006.

25. Simoni JM, Amico KR, Pearson CR, Malow R. Strategies for promoting adherence to anti-retroviral therapy: a review of the literature. Curr Infect Dis Rep. 2008;10(6):515–21. Epub 24 Oct 2008.

26. Simoni JM, Frick PA, Pantalone DW, Turner BJ. Antiretroviral adherence interventions: a review of current literature and ongoing studies. Top HIV Med. 2003;11(6):185–98. Epub 16 Jan 2004.

27. Parienti JJ, Das-Douglas M, Massari V, Guzman D, Deeks SG, Verdon R, et al. Not all missed doses are the same: sustained NNRTI treatment interruptions predict HIV rebound at low-to-moderate adherence levels. PLoS One. 2008;3(7):e2783. Epub 31 July 2008.

28. DiIorio C, McCarty F, Resnicow K, McDonnell Holstad M, Soet J, Yeager K, et al. Using motivational interviewing to promote adherence to antiretroviral medications: a randomized controlled study. AIDS Care. 2008;20(3):273–83. Epub 21 Mar 2008.

29. DiIorio C, Resnicow K, McDonnell M, Soet J, McCarty F, Yeager K. Using motivational interviewing to promote adherence to antiretroviral medications: a pilot study. J Assoc Nurses AIDS Care. 2003;14(2):52–62. Epub 18 Apr 2003.

30. de Bruin M, Viechtbauer W, Hospers HJ, Schaalma HP, Kok G. Standard care quality determines treatment outcomes in control groups of HAART-adherence intervention studies: implications for the interpretation and comparison of intervention effects. Health Psychol. 2009;28(6):668–74. Epub 18 Nov 2009.

31. Amico KR. Standard of care for antiretroviral therapy adherence and retention in care from the perspective of care providers attending the 5th international conference on HIV treatment adherence. J Int Assoc Physicians AIDS Care (Chic). 2011;10(5):291–6. Epub 12 May 2011.

32. Rotheram-Borus MJ, Ingram BL, Swendeman D, Flannery D. Common principles embedded in effective adolescent HIV prevention programs. AIDS Behav. 2009;13(3):387–98. Epub 19 Feb 2009.

33. Rotheram-Borus MJ, Swendeman D, Flannery D, Rice E, Adamson DM, Ingram B. Common factors in effective HIV prevention programs. AIDS Behav. 2009;13(3):399–408. Epub 3 Oct 2008.

34. Ingram BL, Flannery D, Elkavich A, Rotheram-Borus MJ. Common processes in evidence-based adolescent HIV prevention programs. AIDS Behav. 2008;12(3):374–83. Epub 12 Mar 2008.

35. Cassell MM, Halperin DT, Shelton JD, Stanton D. Risk compensation: the Achilles' heel of innovations in HIV prevention? BMJ. 2006;332(7541):605–7. Epub 11 Mar 2006.

36. Phillips KA, Coates TJ. HIV counselling and testing: research and policy issues. AIDS Care. 1995;7(2):115–24. Epub 1 Jan 1995.

37. Bogard E, Kuntz KM. The impact of a partially effective HIV vaccine on a population of intravenous drug users in Bangkok, Thailand: a dynamic model. J Acquir Immune Defic Syndr. 2002;29(2):132–41. Epub 8 Feb 2002.

38. Crosby RA, Holtgrave DR. Will sexual risk behaviour increase after being vaccinated for AIDS? Int J STD AIDS. 2006;17(3):180–4. Epub 3 Mar 2006.

39. Pinkerton SD. Sexual risk compensation and HIV/STD transmission: empirical evidence and theoretical considerations. Risk Anal. 2001;21(4):727–36. Epub 1 Dec 2001.

40. Bailey RC, Moses S, Parker CB, Agot K, Maclean I, Krieger JN, et al. Male circumcision for HIV prevention in young men in Kisumu, Kenya: a randomized controlled trial. Lancet. 2007;369:643–56.

41. Eaton LA, Kalichman SC. Risk compensation in HIV prevention: implications for vaccines, microbicides, and other biomedical HIV prevention technologies. Curr HIV/AIDS Rep. 2007;4:165–72.

42. Kalichman S, Eaton L, Pinkerton S. Circumcision for HIV prevention: failure to fully account for behavioral risk compensation. PLoS Med. 2007;4(3):e138. author reply e46. Epub 29 Mar 2007.

43. Eaton L, Kalichman SC. Behavioral aspects of male circumcision for the prevention of HIV infection. Curr HIV/AIDS Rep. 2009;6(4):187–93. Epub 24 Oct 2009.

44. Abdool Karim Q, Abdool Karim SS, Frohlich JA, Grobler AC, Baxter C, Mansoor LE, et al. Effectiveness and safety of tenofovir gel, an antiretroviral microbicide, for the prevention of HIV infection in women. Science. 2010;329(5996):1168–74. Epub 21 July 2010.

45. Grant RM, Lama JR, Anderson PL, McMahan V, Liu AY, Vargas L, et al. Preexposure chemo-prophylaxis for HIV prevention in men who have sex with men. N Engl J Med. 2010;363(27):2587–99. Epub 26 Nov 2010.

46. Weinhardt LS, Mosack KE, Swain GR. Development of a computer-based risk-reduction counseling intervention: acceptability and preferences among low-income patients at an urban sexually transmitted infection clinic. AIDS Behav. 2007;11(4):549–56. Epub 10 Oct 2006.

47. Grimley DM, Hook 3rd EW. A 15-minute interactive, computerized condom use intervention with biological endpoints. Sex Transm Dis. 2009;36(2):73–8. Epub 7 Jan 2009.

48. Bellis JM, Grimley DM, Alexander LR. Feasibility of a tailored intervention targeting STD-related behaviors. Am J Health Behav. 2002;26(5):378–85. Epub 11 Sept 2002.

49. Fisher JD, Amico KR, Fisher WA, Cornman DH, Shuper PA, Trayling C, et al. Computer-based intervention in HIV clinical care setting improves antiretroviral adherence: the LifeWindows Project. AIDS Behav. 2011;15(8):1635–46. Epub 1 Apr 2011.

50. Reynolds NR, Testa MA, Su M, Chesney MA, Neidig JL, Frank I, et al. Telephone support to improve antiretroviral medication adherence: a multisite, randomized controlled trial. J Acquir Immune Defic Syndr. 2008;47(1):62–8. Epub 25 Sept 2007.

51. Senore C, Giordano L, Bellisario C, Di Stefano F, Segnan N. Population based cancer screening programmes as a teachable moment for primary prevention interventions. A review of the literature. Front Oncol. 2012;2:45. Epub 1 June 2012.

52. McBride CM, Emmons KM, Lipkus IM. Understanding the potential of teachable moments: the case of smoking cessation. Health Educ Res. 2003;18(2):156–70. Epub 6 May 2003.

53. McBride CM, Ostroff JS. Teachable moments for promoting smoking cessation: the context of cancer care and survivorship. Cancer Control. 2003;10(4):325–33. Epub 14 Aug 2003.

54. UNAIDS. Combination HIV prevention: tailoring and coordinating biomedical, behavioural and structural strategies to reduce new HIV infections: a UNAIDS discussion paper. Geneva, Switzerland, 2010.

55. Coates TJ, Richter L, Caceres C. Behavioural strategies to reduce HIV transmission: how to make them work better. Lancet. 2008;372(9639):669–84. Epub 9 Aug 2008.

56. Tatoud RJ. Metaphors of HIV prevention: 1. The HIV prevention buffet. 2011 [cited 2012]. http://www.incidence0.org/2011/05/31/metaphors-of-hiv-prevention-1-the-hiv-prevention-buffet/.

57. Palmateer N, Kimber J, Hickman M, Hutchinson S, Rhodes T, Goldberg D. Evidence for the effectiveness of sterile injecting equipment provision in preventing hepatitis C and human immunodeficiency virus transmission among injecting drug users: a review of reviews. Addiction. 2010;105(5):844–59. Epub 12 Mar 2010.

58. Hyshka E, Strathdee S, Wood E, Kerr T. Needle exchange and the HIV epidemic in Vancouver: lessons learned from 15 years of research. Int J Drug Policy. 2012. Epub 15 May 2012.

59. Gillies M, Palmateer N, Hutchinson S, Ahmed S, Taylor A, Goldberg D. The provision of non-needle/syringe drug injecting paraphernalia in the primary prevention of HCV among IDU: a systematic review. BMC Public Health. 2010;10:721. Epub 26 Nov 2010.

60. Kalichman SC, Kelly JA, Sikkema KJ, Koslov AP, Shaboltas A, Granskaya J. The emerging AIDS crisis in Russia: review of enabling factors and prevention needs. Int J STD AIDS. 2000;11(2):71–5. Epub 4 Mar 2000.

61. Tobin KE, Muessig KE, Latkin CA. HIV seropositive drug users' attitudes towards partner notification (PCRS): results from the SHIELD study in Baltimore, Maryland. Patient Educ Couns. 2007;67(1–2):137–42. Epub 24 Apr 2007.

62. Latkin CA, Sherman S, Knowlton A. HIV prevention among drug users: outcome of a network-oriented peer outreach intervention. Health Psychol. 2003;22(4):332–9. Epub 28 Aug 2003.

63. Purcell DW, Metsch LR, Latka M, Santibanez S, Gomez CA, Eldred L, et al. Interventions for seropositive injectors-research and evaluation: an integrated behavioral intervention with HIV-positive injection drug users to address medical care, adherence, and risk reduction. J Acquir Immune Defic Syndr. 2004;37 Suppl 2:S110–8. Epub 24 Sept 2004.

64. Knowlton AR, Hua W, Latkin C. Social support networks and medical service use among HIV-positive injection drug users: implications to intervention. AIDS Care. 2005;17(4):479–92. Epub 23 July 2005.

65. Latkin CA, Donnell D, Metzger D, Sherman S, Aramrattna A, Davis-Vogel A, et al. The efficacy of a network intervention to reduce HIV risk behaviors among drug users and risk partners in Chiang Mai, Thailand and Philadelphia, USA. Soc Sci Med. 2009;68(4):740–8. Epub 17 Dec 2008.

66. Tobin KE, Hua W, Costenbader EC, Latkin CA. The association between change in social network characteristics and non-fatal overdose: results from the SHIELD study in Baltimore, MD, USA. Drug Alcohol Depend. 2007;87(1):63–8. Epub 12 Sept 2006.

67. Latkin CA, Davey MA, Hua W. Social context of needle selling in Baltimore, Maryland. Subst Use Misuse. 2006;41(6–7):901–13. Epub 1 July 2006.

68. Friedman SR, Bolyard M, Mateu-Gelabert P, Goltzman P, Pawlowicz MP, Singh DZ, et al. Some data-driven reflections on priorities in AIDS network research. AIDS Behav. 2007;11(5):641–51. Epub 21 Oct 2006.

69. Friedman SR, Mateu-Gelabert P, Curtis R, Maslow C, Bolyard M, Sandoval M, et al. Social capital or networks, negotiations, and norms? A neighborhood case study. Am J Prev Med. 2007;32(6 Suppl):S160–70. Epub 19 Aug 2007.

70. Kost K, Singh S, Vaughan B, Trussell J, Bankole A. Estimates of contraceptive failure from the 2002 National Survey of Family Growth. Contraception. 2008;77(1):10–21. Epub 18 Dec 2007.
71. Crosby RA, Diclemente RJ, Wingood GM, Salazar LF, Rose E, Levine D, et al. Correlates of condom failure among adolescent males: an exploratory study. Prev Med. 2005;41(5–6):873–6. Epub 1 Nov 2005.
72. Kalichman SC, Simbayi LC, Cain D, Jooste S. Condom failure among men receiving sexually transmissible infection clinic services, Cape Town, South Africa. Sex Health. 2009;6(4):300–4. Epub 18 Nov 2009.
73. Chow EP, Wilson DP, Zhang L. Patterns of condom use among men who have sex with men in China: a systematic review and meta-analysis. AIDS Behav. 2012;16(3):653–63. Epub 5 Apr 2011.
74. Kelly JA, Kalichman SC. Increased attention to human sexuality can improve HIV-AIDS prevention efforts: key research issues and directions. J Consult Clin Psychol. 1995;63(6):907–18. Epub 1 Dec 1995.
75. Koop CE. The early days of AIDS, as I remember them. Ann Forum Collab HIV Res. 2011;13:5–10.
76. Trenholm C, Devaney B, Fortson K, Clark M, Bridgespan LQ, Wheeler J. Impacts of abstinence education on teen sexual activity, risk of pregnancy, and risk of sexually transmitted diseases. J Policy Anal Manage. 2008;27(2):255–76. Epub 12 Apr 2008.
77. Jemmott 3rd JB, Jemmott LS, Fong GT. Abstinence and safer sex HIV risk-reduction interventions for African American adolescents: a randomized controlled trial. JAMA. 1998;279(19):1529–36. Epub 30 May 1998.
78. Barnett T, Parkhurst J. HIV/AIDS: sex, abstinence, and behaviour change. Lancet Infect Dis. 2005;5(9):590–3. Epub 27 Aug 2005.
79. Lyles CM, Kay LS, Crepaz N, Herbst JH, Passin WF, Kim AS, et al. Best-evidence interventions: findings from a systematic review of HIV behavioral interventions for US populations at high risk, 2000-2004. Am J Public Health. 2007;97(1):133–43. Epub 2 Dec 2006.
80. Nelson KE, Celentano DD, Eiumtrakol S, Hoover DR, Beyrer C, Suprasert S, et al. Changes in sexual behavior and a decline in HIV infection among young men in Thailand. N Engl J Med. 1996;335(5):297–303. Epub 1 Aug 1996.
81. Rojanapithayakorn W, Hanenberg R. The 100% condom program in Thailand. AIDS. 1996;10(1):1–7. Epub 1 Jan 1996.
82. National Institutes of Health. NIH Consensus Statement: Interventions to Prevent HIV Risk Behavior. 15(2), February 11–13, 1997. Available at http://consensus.nih.gov/1997/1997PreventHIVRisk104PDF.pdf.
83. Wingood GM, DiClemente RJ, Mikhail I, Lang DL, McCree DH, Davies SL, et al. A randomized controlled trial to reduce HIV transmission risk behaviors and sexually transmitted diseases among women living with HIV: The WiLLOW Program. J Acquir Immune Defic Syndr. 2004;37 Suppl 2:S58–67. Epub 24 Sept 2004.
84. Sandoy IF, Zyaambo C, Michelo C, Fylkesnes K. Targeting condom distribution at high risk places increases condom utilization-evidence from an intervention study in Livingstone, Zambia. BMC Public Health. 2012;12:10. Epub 10 Jan 2012.
85. Kenya: Female Condom Shortage. Humanitarian news and analysis. 2009.
86. Cecil H, Pinkerton SD, Bogart LM. Perceived benefits and barriers associated with the female condom among African-American adults. J Health Psychol. 1999;4(2):165–75. Epub 1 Mar 1999.
87. Gallo MF, Kilbourne-Brook M, Coffey PS. A review of the effectiveness and acceptability of the female condom for dual protection. Sex Health. 2012;9(1):18–26. Epub 22 Feb 2012.
88. Beksinska ME, Smit JA, Mantell JE. Progress and challenges to male and female condom use in South Africa. Sex Health. 2012;9(1):51–8. Epub 22 Feb 2012.
89. Kelvin EA, Mantell JE, Candelario N, Hoffman S, Exner TM, Stackhouse W, et al. Off-label use of the female condom for anal intercourse among men in New York City. Am J Public Health. 2011;101(12):2241–4. Epub 25 Oct 2011.

90. Kalichman SC, Rompa D, Cage M. Factors associated with female condom use among HIV-seropositive women. Int J STD AIDS. 2000;11(12):798–803. Epub 4 Jan 2001.

91. Marseille E, Kahn JG. Smarter programming of the female condom: increasing its impact on HIV prevention in the developing world. Published by FSG Social Impact Advisors, Available at http://www.fsg.org/Portals/0/Uploads/Documents/PDF/Female_Condom_Impact.pdf.

92. Kalichman SC, Williams E, Nachimson D. Brief behavioural skills building intervention for female controlled methods of STD-HIV prevention: outcomes of a randomized clinical field trial. Int J STD AIDS. 1999;10(3):174–81. Epub 26 May 1999.

93. Hoke TH, Feldblum PJ, Damme KV, Nasution MD, Grey TW, Wong EL, et al. Randomised controlled trial of alternative male and female condom promotion strategies targeting sex workers in Madagascar. Sex Transm Infect. 2007;83(6):448–53. Epub 27 June 2007.

94. Marks G, Crepaz N, Janssen RS. Estimating sexual transmission of HIV from persons aware and unaware that they are infected with the virus in the USA. AIDS. 2006;20(10):1447–50. Epub 23 June 2006.

95. Phillips KA, Bayer R, Chen JL. New Centers for Disease Control and Prevention's guidelines on HIV counseling and testing for the general population and pregnant women. J Acquir Immune Defic Syndr. 2003;32(2):182–91. Epub 7 Feb 2003.

96. Holtgrave D, McGuire J. Impact of counseling in voluntary counseling and testing programs for persons at risk for or living with HIV infection. Clin Infect Dis. 2007;45 Suppl 4:S240–3. Epub 8 Feb 2008.

97. Estrada BD, Trujillo S, Estrada AL. Supporting Healthy Alternatives through Patient Education: a theoretically driven HIV prevention intervention for persons living with HIV/AIDS. AIDS Behav. 2007;11(5 Suppl):S95–105. Epub 1 Feb 2007.

98. Metcalf CA, Malotte CK, Douglas Jr JM, Paul SM, Dillon BA, Cross H, et al. Efficacy of a booster counseling session 6 months after HIV testing and counseling: a randomized, controlled trial (RESPECT-2). Sex Transm Dis. 2005;32(2):123–9. Epub 26 Jan 2005.

99. Cohen MS, Shaw GM, McMichael AJ, Haynes BF. Acute HIV-1 infection. N Engl J Med. 2011;364(20):1943–54. Epub 20 May 2011.

100. Hightow-Weidman LB, Golin CE, Green K, Shaw EN, MacDonald PD, Leone PA. Identifying people with acute HIV infection: demographic features, risk factors, and use of health care among individuals with AHI in North Carolina. AIDS Behav. 2009;13(6):1075–83. Epub 8 Jan 2009.

101. Kelly JA, St Lawrence JS, Diaz YE, Stevenson LY, Hauth AC, Brasfield TL, et al. HIV risk behavior reduction following intervention with key opinion leaders of population: an experimental analysis. Am J Public Health. 1991;81(2):168–71. Epub 1 Feb 1991.

102. Kelly JA, St Lawrence JS, Stevenson LY, Hauth AC, Kalichman SC, Diaz YE, et al. Community AIDS/HIV risk reduction: the effects of endorsements by popular people in three cities. Am J Public Health. 1992;82(11):1483–9 Epub 1 Nov 1992.

103. Kelly JA, Murphy DA, Sikkema KJ, McAuliffe TL, Roffman RA, Solomon LJ, et al. Randomised, controlled, community-level HIV-prevention intervention for sexual-risk behaviour among homosexual men in US cities. Community HIV Prevention Research Collaborative. Lancet. 1997;350(9090):1500–5. Epub 6 Dec 1997.

104. Morin SF. AIDS: the challenge to psychology. Am Psychol. 1988;43(11):838–42. Epub 1 Nov 1988.

105. Connor EM, Sperling RS, Gelber R, Kiselev P, Scott G, O'Sullivan MJ, et al. Reduction of maternal-infant transmission of human immunodeficiency virus type 1 with zidovudine treatment. Pediatric AIDS Clinical Trials Group Protocol 076 Study Group. N Engl J Med. 1994;331(18):1173–80. Epub 3 Nov 1994.

106. Trust NA. HIV treatment as prevention. UK: National AIDS Trust; 2011.

107. Padian NS. Sexual histories of heterosexual couples with one HIV-infected partner. Am J Public Health. 1990;80(8):990–1. Epub 1 Aug 1990.

108. Cohen MS, Hoffman IF, Royce RA, Kazembe P, Dyer JR, Daly CC, et al. Reduction of concentration of HIV-1 in semen after treatment of urethritis: implications for prevention of

sexual transmission of HIV-1. AIDSCAP Malawi Research Group. Lancet. 1997;349(9069):1868–73. Epub 28 June 1997.

109. Steward WT, Remien RH, Higgins JA, Dubrow R, Pinkerton SD, Sikkema KJ, et al. Behavior change following diagnosis with acute/early HIV infection—a move to serosorting with other HIV-infected individuals. The NIMH Multisite Acute HIV Infection Study: III. AIDS Behav. 2009;13(6):1054–60. Epub 9 June 2009.

110. Wawer MJ, Gray RH, Sewankarnbo NK, Serwadda D, Li X, Laeyendecker O, et al. Rates of HIV-1 transmission per coital act, by stage of HIV-1 infection, in Rakai, Uganda. J Infect Dis. 2005;191(9):1403–9.

111. Mehta SD, Gray RH, Auvert B, Moses S, Kigozi G, Taljaard D, et al. Does sex in the early period after circumcision increase HIV-seroconversion risk? Pooled analysis of adult male circumcision clinical trials. AIDS. 2009;23(12):1557–64. Epub 3 July 2009.

112. Cohen MS, Hosseinipour M. HIV treatment meets prevention: antiretroviral therapy as prophylaxis. In: M P, editor. The AIDS pandemic: impact on science and society. New York: Elsevier; 2004.

113. Kalichman SC, Simbayi LC. Sexual exposure to blood and behavioural risks among STI clinic patients in Cape Town, South Africa. Sex Health. 2005;2(2):85–8. Epub 14 Dec 2005.

114. Kalichman SC, Simbayi LC, Cain D, Cherry C, Jooste S. Coital bleeding and HIV risks among men and women in Cape Town, South Africa. Sex Transm Dis. 2006;33(9):551–7. Epub 12 May 2006.

115. Kalichman SC, Cain D, Simbayi LC. Behavioral changes associated with testing HIV-positive among sexually transmitted infection clinic patients in Cape Town, South Africa. Am J Public Health. 2010;100(4):714–9. Epub 20 Feb 2010.

116. Boily MC, Baggaley RF, Wang L, Masse B, White RG, Hayes RJ, et al. Heterosexual risk of HIV-1 infection per sexual act: systematic review and meta-analysis of observational studies. Lancet Infect Dis. 2009;9(2):118–29. Epub 31 Jan 2009.

117. Powers KA, Ghani AC, Miller WC, Hoffman IF, Pettifor AE, Kamanga G, et al. The role of acute and early HIV infection in the spread of HIV and implications for transmission prevention strategies in Lilongwe, Malawi: a modelling study. Lancet. 2011;378(9787):256–68. Epub 21 June 2011.

118. Coates TJ, Stall RD, Catania JA, Kegeles SM. Behavioral factors in the spread of HIV infection. AIDS. 1988;2 Suppl 1:S239–46. Epub 1 Jan 1988.

119. Stall RD, Coates TJ, Hoff C. Behavioral risk reduction for HIV infection among gay and bisexual men. A review of results from the United States. Am Psychol. 1988;43(11):878–85. Epub 1 Nov 1988.

120. Lescano CM, Houck CD, Brown LK, Doherty G, DiClemente RJ, Fernandez MI, et al. Correlates of heterosexual anal intercourse among at-risk adolescents and young adults. Am J Public Health. 2009;99(6):1131–6. Epub 15 Nov 2008.

121. Mosher WD, Chandra A, Jones J. Sexual behavior and selected health measures: men and women 15–44 years of age, United States, 2002. Adv Data. 2005;362:1–55. Epub 28 Oct 2005.

122. Kalichman SC, Simbayi LC, Cain D, Jooste S. Heterosexual anal intercourse among community and clinical settings in Cape Town, South Africa. Sex Transm Infect. 2009;85(6):411–5. Epub 12 May 2009.

123. Kalichman SC, Pinkerton SD, Carey MP, Cain D, Mehlomakulu V, Carey KB, et al. Heterosexual anal intercourse and HIV infection risks in the context of alcohol serving venues, Cape Town, South Africa. BMC Public Health. 2011;11:807. Epub 18 Oct 2011.

124. Fang CT, Hsu HM, Twu SJ, Chen MY, Chang YY, Hwang JS, et al. Decreased HIV transmission after a policy of providing free access to highly active antiretroviral therapy in Taiwan. J Infect Dis. 2004;190(5):879–85. Epub 6 Aug 2004.

125. Baeten JM, Kahle E, Lingappa JR, Coombs RW, Delany-Moretlwe S, Nakku-Joloba E, et al. Genital HIV-1 RNA predicts risk of heterosexual HIV-1 transmission. Sci Transl Med. 2011;3(77):77ra29. Epub 8 Apr 2011.

126. Pao D, Pillay D, Fisher M. Potential impact of early antiretroviral therapy on transmission. Curr Opin HIV AIDS. 2009;4(3):215–21. Epub 18 June 2009.

127. Attia S, Egger M, Muller M, Zwahlen M, Low N. Sexual transmission of HIV according to viral load and antiretroviral therapy: systematic review and meta-analysis. AIDS. 2009;23(11):1397–404. Epub 22 Apr 2009.
128. Hull MW, Montaner J. Antiretroviral therapy: a key component of a comprehensive HIV prevention strategy. Curr HIV/AIDS Rep. 2011;8(2):85–93. Epub 30 Mar 2011.
129. Smith K, Powers KA, Kashuba AD, Cohen MS. HIV-1 treatment as prevention: the good, the bad, and the challenges. Curr Opin HIV AIDS. 2011;6(4):315–25. Epub 8 June 2011.
130. Cowan SA, Gerstoft J, Haff J, Hartvig Christiansen A, Statistician JN, Obel N. Stable incidence of HIV diagnoses among Danish MSM despite increased engagement in unsafe sex. J Acquir Immune Defic Syndr. 2012. Epub 18 May 2012.
131. Jin F, Jansson J, Law M, Prestage GP, Zablotska I, Imrie JC, et al. Per-contact probability of HIV transmission in homosexual men in Sydney in the era of HAART. AIDS. 2010;24(6): 907–13. Epub 9 Feb 2010.
132. Granich RM, Gilks CF, Dye C, De Cock KM, Williams BG. Universal voluntary HIV testing with immediate antiretroviral therapy as a strategy for elimination of HIV transmission: a mathematical model. Lancet. 2009;373(9657):48–57. Epub 29 Nov 2008.
133. Dieffenbach CW, Fauci AS. Universal voluntary testing and treatment for prevention of HIV transmission. JAMA. 2009;301(22):2380–2. Epub 11 June 2009.
134. Hallett TB, Smit C, Garnett GP, de Wolf F. Estimating the risk of HIV transmission from homosexual men receiving treatment to their HIV-uninfected partners. Sex Transm Infect. 2011;87(1):17–21. Epub 21 July 2010.
135. Cohen MS, McCauley M, Gamble TR. HIV treatment as prevention and HPTN 052. Curr Opin HIV AIDS. 2012;7(2):99–105. Epub 10 Jan 2012.
136. Cohen MS, Chen YQ, McCauley M, Gamble T, Hosseinipour MC, Kumarasamy N, et al. Prevention of HIV-1 infection with early antiretroviral therapy. N Engl J Med. 2011;365(6):493–505. Epub 20 July 2011.
137. Cohen MS, Gay CL. Treatment to prevent transmission of HIV-1. Clin Infect Dis. 2010;50 Suppl 3:S85–95. Epub 20 Apr 2010.
138. Vernazza PL, Eron JJ, Cohen MS, van der Horst CM, Troiani L, Fiscus SA. Detection and biologic characterization of infectious HIV-1 in semen of seropositive men. AIDS. 1994;8(9):1325–9. Epub 1 Sept 1994.
139. Vernazza PL, Gilliam BL, Flepp M, Dyer JR, Frank AC, Fiscus SA, et al. Effect of antiviral treatment on the shedding of HIV-1 in semen. AIDS. 1997;11(10):1249–54. Epub 1 Aug 1997.
140. Vernazza PL, Troiani L, Flepp MJ, Cone RW, Schock J, Roth F, et al. Potent antiretroviral treatment of HIV infection results in suppression of the seminal shedding of HIV. AIDS. 2000;14(2):117–21.
141. Vernazza P, Hirschel B, Bernasconi E, Flepp M. HIV-positive individuals without additional sexually transmitted diseases (STD) and on effective anti-retroviral therapy are sexually non-infectious. Bulletin des médecins suisses 2008;89(5):165–9.
142. Strub S. Swiss say condoms not necessary…sometimes. Huffington Post, March 26, 2008. Available at http://www.huffingtonpost.com/sean-strub/swiss-say-condoms-not-nec_b_93574.html.
143. WHO-UNAIDS. Antiretroviral therapy and sexual transmission of HIV. UNAIDS, Geneva, Switzerland. Available at http://data.unaids.org/pub/pressstatement/2008/080201_hivtransmission_en.pdf.
144. Pinkerton SD. How many sexually-acquired HIV infections in the USA are due to acute-phase HIV transmission? AIDS. 2007;21(12):1625–9. Epub 17 July 2007.
145. Cohen MS. HIV treatment as prevention and "the Swiss statement": in for a dime, in for a dollar? Clin Infect Dis. 2010;51(11):1323–4. Epub 3 Nov 2010.
146. Kalichman SC, Di Berto G, Eaton L. Human immunodeficiency virus viral load in blood plasma and semen: review and implications of empirical findings. Sex Transm Dis. 2008;35(1):55–60. Epub 25 Jan 2008.

147. Hosein S, Wilson D. Decision-making by people living with HIV requires communication from clinicians about the risks of transmission despite undetectable plasma viral load. HIV Med. 2010;12:516.

148. Kalichman SC, Cage M, Barnett T, Tharnish P, Rompa D, Austin J, et al. Human immunodeficiency virus in semen and plasma: investigation of sexual transmission risk behavioral correlates. AIDS Res Hum Retroviruses. 2001;17(18):1695–703. Epub 15 Jan 2002.

149. Cu-Uvin S, Hogan JW, Caliendo AM, Harwell J, Mayer KH, Carpenter CC. Association between bacterial vaginosis and expression of human immunodeficiency virus type 1 RNA in the female genital tract. Clin Infect Dis. 2001;33(6):894–6. Epub 21 Aug 2001.

150. Vernazza P, Kashuba A, Cohen MS. Biological correlates of sexual transmission of HIV: practical consequences and potential targets for public health. Rev Med Microbiol. 2001;12(3):131–42.

151. Reichelderfer PS, Coombs RW, Wright DJ, Cohn J, Burns DN, Cu-Uvin S, et al. Effect of menstrual cycle on HIV-1 levels in the peripheral blood and genital tract WHS 001 Study Team. AIDS. 2000;14(14):2101–7. Epub 4 Nov 2000.

152. Kalichman SC, Eaton L, Cherry C. Sexually transmitted infections and infectiousness beliefs among people living with HIV/AIDS: implications for HIV treatment as prevention. HIV Med. 2010;11(8):502–9. Epub 6 Mar 2010.

153. Kalichman SC, Rompa D, Austin J, Luke W, DiFonzo K. Viral load, perceived infectivity, and unprotected intercourse. J Acquir Immune Defic Syndr. 2001;28(3):303–5. Epub 6 Nov 2001.

154. Hasse B, Ledergerber B, Hirschel B, Vernazza P, Glass TR, Jeannin A, et al. Frequency and determinants of unprotected sex among HIV-infected persons: the Swiss HIV cohort study. Clin Infect Dis. 2010;51(11):1314–22. Epub 3 Nov 2010.

155. Johnson LF, Lewis DA. The effect of genital tract infections on HIV-1 shedding in the genital tract: a systematic review and meta-analysis. Sex Transm Dis. 2008;35(11):946–59. Epub 8 Aug 2008.

156. Kalichman SC, Pellowski J, Turner C. Prevalence of sexually transmitted co-infections in people living with HIV/AIDS: systematic review with implications for using HIV treatments for prevention. Sex Transm Infect. 2011;87(3):183–90. Epub 19 Feb 2011.

157. Holtgrave DR, Maulsby C, Wehrmeyer L, Hall HI. Behavioral factors in assessing impact of HIV treatment as prevention. AIDS Behav. 2012;16(5):1085–91. Epub 12 Apr 2012.

158. Holtgrave DR, Hall HI, Wehrmeyer L, Maulsby C. Costs, consequences and feasibility of strategies for achieving the goals of the National HIV/AIDS Strategy in the United States: a closing window for success? AIDS Behav. 2012. Epub 23 May 2012.

159. Kurth AE, McClelland L, Wanje G, Ghee AE, Peshu N, Mutunga E, et al. An integrated approach for antiretroviral adherence and secondary HIV transmission risk-reduction support by nurses in Kenya. J Assoc Nurses AIDS Care. 2012;23(2):146–54. Epub 2 Aug 2011.

160. Ewart C. Social action theory for a public health psychology. Am Psychol. 1991;465:931–46.

161. Ewart C. How integrative behavioral theory can improve health promotion and disease prevention. In: Boll TJ, Frank RG, Baum A, Wallander J, editors. Handbook of health psychology. Washington, DC: American Psychological Association; 2004.

162. Gore-Felton C, Rotheram-Borus MJ, Weinhardt LS, Kelly JA, Lightfoot M, Kirshenbaum SB, et al. The Healthy Living Project: an individually tailored, multidimensional intervention for HIV-infected persons. AIDS Educ Prev. 2005;17(1 Suppl A):21–39. Epub 22 Apr 2005.

163. Chesney MA, Chambers DB, Taylor JM, Johnson LM, Folkman S. Coping effectiveness training for men living with HIV: results from a randomized clinical trial testing a group-based intervention. Psychosom Med. 2003;65(6):1038–46. Epub 4 Dec 2003.

164. Chesney M, Folkman S, Chambers D. Coping effectiveness training for men living with HIV: preliminary findings. Int J STD AIDS. 1996;7 Suppl 2:75–82. Epub 1 Jan 1996.

165. Healthy Living Project Team. Effects of a behavioral intervention to reduce risk of transmission among people living with HIV: the healthy living project randomized controlled study. J Acquir Immune Defic Syndr. 2007;44(2):213–21. Epub 6 Dec 2006.

166. Johnson MO, Charlebois E, Morin SF, Remien RH, Chesney MA. Effects of a behavioral intervention on antiretroviral medication adherence among people living with HIV: the healthy living project randomized controlled study. J Acquir Immune Defic Syndr. 2007;46(5):574–80. Epub 15 Jan 2008.

167. Pinkerton SD, Holtgrave DR, Valdiserri RO. Cost-effectiveness of HIV-prevention skills training for men who have sex with men. AIDS. 1997;11(3):347–57. Epub 1 Mar 1997.

168. Pinkerton SD, Holtgrave DR. How HIV treatment advances affect the cost-effectiveness of prevention. Med Decis Making. 2000;20(1):89–94. Epub 19 Jan 2000.

169. Prochaska JO, Velicer WF. The transtheoretical model of health behavior change. Am J Health Promot. 1997;12(1):38–48. Epub 5 Aug 1997.

170. Miller WR, Rose GS. Toward a theory of motivational interviewing. Am Psychol. 2009;64(6):527–37. Epub 11 Sept 2009.

171. Holstad M, DiIorio C, Magowe M. Motivating HIV positive women to adhere to antiretroviral therapy and risk reduction behavior: The KHARMA Project. J Issues Nurs. 2006; 11:1–19.

172. Holstad MM, DiIorio C, Kelley ME, Resnicow K, Sharma S. Group motivational interviewing to promote adherence to antiretroviral medications and risk reduction behaviors in HIV infected women. AIDS Behav. 2011;15(5):885–96. Epub 18 Nov 2010.

173. Kalichman SC, Cherry C, Kalichman MO, Amaral CM, White D, Pope H, et al. Integrated behavioral intervention to improve HIV/AIDS treatment adherence and reduce HIV transmission. Am J Public Health. 2011;101(3):531–8. Epub 15 Jan 2011.

174. Des Jarlais DC, Perlis T, Arasteh K, Torian LV, Hagan H, Beatrice S, et al. HIV incidence among injection drug users in New York City, 1990 to 2002: Use of serologic test algorithm to assess expansion of HIV prevention services. Am J Public Health. 2005;95(8): 1439–1445.

# Index